CONFESSIONS
of a
Surly Barber

CONFESSIONS
of a
Surly Barber

Increasing the Odds of
Getting a Great Haircut

Mara Stewart

iUniverse, Inc.
New York Lincoln Shanghai

CONFESSIONS of a Surly Barber
Increasing the Odds of Getting a Great Haircut

iUniverse books may be ordered through booksellers or by contacting:

iUniverse
2021 Pine Lake Road, Suite 100
Lincoln, NE 68512
www.iuniverse.com
1-800-Authors (1-800-288-4677)

The views expressed in this work are solely those of the author and do not necessarily reflect the views of the publisher, and the publisher hereby disclaims any responsibility for them.

ISBN-13: 978-0-595-42317-0 (pbk)
ISBN-13: 978-0-595-86656-4 (ebk)
ISBN-10: 0-595-42317-5 (pbk)
ISBN-10: 0-595-86656-5 (ebk)

Printed in the United States of America

THIS BOOK IS DEDICATED TO MY DAUGHTER,
CASSIE

Table Of Contents

The Circle Of Life

Confessions

Surly (adjective)

1) *given to or displaying a resentful silence and often irritability <went about his chores in a surly huff, totally annoyed that he was stuck at home on this beautiful Saturday>*

2) *having or showing a habitually bad temper< the surly receptionist told us we'd have to wait outside in the rain>*

Surly (Synonym)

disagreeable, hostile, antagonistic, sulky, ill-tempered

Introduction

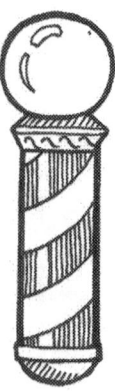

Acknowledgments

I would like to express thanks to the following friends and family for their vital part in transforming the manuscript into this book, for their editorial help and never ending praise and encouragement.

My love and deep gratitude to my mother, Mary Hyatt, who always believes in me and has always inspired me by her example. She has helped immensely from start to finish always providing encouragement and editorial help.

Heartfelt thanks to my good friends Leigh Ann Cheek and Suzanne Doucette. They both put up with me through it all and read the book as I was writing it, giving me encouragement, correcting my grammar and helping me along with everything, every step of the way, from the initial idea to the final editing. I couldn't have finished the book without their help.

Many thanks to my friend SueAnn Landes, whom I met in the barber shop as a customer, then later became my friend and mentor. The universe works in mysterious ways.

Another customer who became a friend over the years, I'd like to thank Jimmy Green for his support, feedback and editorial assistance.

I would like to thank all the barbers I've worked along with while I've been writing this book. They answered questions and discussed the issues related to the book with me. I couldn't have done it without them. Special thanks to Lisa Nandhavan and Dorothy Connell for their additional editorial help. And to Don Andres for taking the time to read the manuscript before publication and offer me his opinion. I put a lot of value in his opinion as a traditional barber from the "old school."

I'd also like to thank Jim McFarland for taking the time to read the manuscript before publication and offer me his opinion and encouragement. As a fellow barber who knew nothing about the book before reading it, I valued his feedback.

Also to Robin and Nick Marfione who own and operate a hairstyling salon next door to my barber shop, for their help all along the way and opinions and feedback.

Heartfelt thanks to my book's artist, Ellen Lyons Harris, for all the illustrations. She took the time to read the text and gave her illustrations the character that makes the book what it is. I am very grateful to have her on board.

I would like to express my gratitude to my sister, Holly VanSickle, for having the guts to go to barber school, and being the pioneer in my family, which I and my three sisters followed. There is no telling what I would be doing for a living right now if it weren't for her having gone first.

Finally I would like to thank the customers. I am grateful to have shared in the lives of so many wonderful people.

Hair's My Story

At the time of this writing, I've been a barber for twenty six years. I attended Miami Barber College, which was later re-named Roffler School Of Hair Design in Ft. Lauderdale, Florida when I was sixteen years old, in 1980. It was an uncommon vocation for women when I first started, as barbers (in America) were usually men. With the exception of my very first job, I've always worked in old-fashioned, traditional barber shops.

People often ask me why I became a barber. Sometimes they just want to know why I became interested in the hair business, and sometimes they want to know why I became a barber, as opposed to becoming a hairstylist/cosmetologist. To be honest, I never thought of doing hair or cutting hair at all during my childhood. Much less did I ever think of becoming a *barber*.

As a child, I spent my youth riding horseback, playing in the woods, and working with my father, who was a large animal veterinarian. I guess I thought I was going to be a veterinarian or a jockey when I grew up. At any rate, becoming a barber was not something I had planned for.

My older sister, Holly became interested in hair-cutting when she was in High School. She got a summer job in a barber shop sweeping the floor and answering the telephone. The shop where she worked had both barbers and cosmetologists working in it. She watched them working and decided she wanted to go to school to learn the trade. She was more interested in cutting the hair than fixing it up, so they all thought she would like barber school more than cosmetology school. She did some research and decided to go to a barber school in Orlando, Florida.

When I finished high school, Holly was working as a barber, doing quite well, and she liked what she was doing. Having no interest in going to college, and not having a clue as to what I wanted to do with my life, my mother insisted that I learn a trade or skill of some sort. So I agreed to try out barber school too. My mom brought me to the barber school in Fort Lauderdale, Florida and before I knew it, I was enrolled there. I don't remember having a whole lot to say in the matter, but it sounded exciting to be on my own in a big city. She bought a car for me and rented an apartment for me not far from the school. There is a law that one must be at least seventeen years of age to take the barber state board exam, but I would be turning seventeen before the time I would graduate, so it was ok.

I was the youngest student there. In Florida, at the time I went to school, it was required to attend for fifteen hundred hours. It took me about eight months to finish school, putting in forty hours per week. I met some wonderful people and made some good friends. It was a lot of fun too. I graduated, took the state board exam and received my licence in September of 1981.

Moving back home, I went looking for employment with my new skill. In 1981, there weren't many female barbers around. There was a time in history that female barbers were unheard of. Having no experience, being young, and not looking the part, I was rejected by each of the barber shops I went to. At that time, there were five or six barber shops in town. I became very discouraged, and finally decided to try the hairstyling salons. I got a job and started right away. It wasn't at all what I wanted to be doing and I didn't like the lady I worked for at all. She didn't seem to like me all that much either. Many days I went home in tears. I had made some good friends in barber school and I had kept in touch with a girl who had graduated and took her state board test around the same time as me. She was from a family of Italian barbers from New York who owned a barber shop in Delray Beach. She suggested I relocate and work with her. Her uncle's shop was really busy and she assured me that I would make good money there. So I moved back to that area and worked there with her.

Her uncle had many years of experience, and was a very good barber. He took me under his wing and taught me what he knew, which was completely different than what I had learned in barber school. I learned so much from him, and will be forever grateful for his kindness. Those folks were great people and I worked there for a several years.

While I was there, my fiancé decided to go to barber school. Making more money than I ever imagined I would be making, it was no problem for me to keep things going while he quit his job and went to school. He enrolled in the Roffler Barber School in West Palm Beach. About a year later, he graduated and got his license. He got a job right away and we were doing quite well.

We were married when I was twenty years old, in 1984. Sometimes I would go visit with him at the school while he was a student. The other students and teachers learned that I was a barber. We became friends with one of the teachers and his wife. One day his teacher asked me if I would be interested in teaching at the school. I had never given it a thought, but it sounded like fun. I decided to try it. The students were required to call me Mrs. Stewart, which was really funny because I was younger than any of my students, and I wasn't used to my new last name yet. I learned more from teaching than I could have imagined. It was a highly rewarding job. I worked there full time (day shift) for two years. I also worked there part time (evenings) as a second job over the next three years.

My husband and I decided to buy a barber shop that was for sale in West Palm Beach. We didn't know the area well and didn't research anything before jumping in with both feet. We borrowed the money from my dad and signed a lease for a five year term with the landlord. It ended up being in a really bad, high crime area of town. It was in downtown West Palm Beach, on Clematis Street, which has since become a very desirable area. We were burglarized twice in the first year. One time, we had to go to the shop in the middle of the night and had to stay there until we could get a glass company to come in the morning to repair the shattered door. That was scary.

We weren't making ends meet either. We were used to making good money, but we were struggling with our own place. That's why I was working a second job in the evenings teaching at the barber school. My husband was working during the day at another barber shop to bring in more money, while I was working at our shop alone by myself. We had bitten off more than we could chew. I was robbed at knife point one day and had the daylights scared out of me so we decided to sell the place.

We were in a bad area and the shop was not making enough money to cover itself, much less our personal expenses, so it was one thing to say we wanted to sell it and quite another thing to actually find someone to sell it to. The percentage of people in the world looking to buy a barber shop anywhere is quite a small number. We couldn't just close up and walk away because we were legally obligated to a five year lease and we had a loan to pay back. We were stuck for quite a while but we finally sold it for just enough to pay back the remainder of the loan and get out of the lease. Then we were free at last. We moved back home and both of us got jobs.

In 1988, my husband and I decided to try it again. We bought another barber shop, but this time we knew the area well. Our second shop was a much better investment. We did well. We remodeled it and built the business up. We were there four years at which time we split up and divorced.

My former husband stayed there and I got a job somewhere else. I stayed at that job for ten years, and then I moved to Maryland and got a job at a barber shop there. I worked for a man there who was from the Philippines. All the barbers in that shop were from Asian countries. Their techniques of barbering were completely different from what I knew and I learned a lot from them. One thing I learned was "When in Rome, do as the Romans do." The shop wasn't far from Washington DC and there were a lot of military bases nearby. The haircuts were much shorter than I was used to. The "skin fade" haircut was very popular there at the time, and it was all new to me. I had to learn how to do it from watching the other barbers. Sometimes you have to fake like you know what you're doing. You have to walk the walk until you can talk the talk. Two years later, I moved back home to Florida and found a job there. After a year and a half my boss asked if I wanted to buy the shop. I bought it in October 2003 and then remodeled it the following month. It is where I am working presently.

Preface

Over the years, I've worked with many talented barbers. I've learned a lot from each of them. Being a barber school instructor was a great experience for me. Experience is everything in this business. The more practice you get, the better your skills become. I'm still learning new things. You learn techniques and tricks from your co-workers. You see many different ways of handling a variety of situations. We talk about the things we like about our business and we also talk to each other about all the things that customers do that drive us nuts. Dealing with these situations day after day for so many years, I found myself becoming "surly" at times. At some point, I started joking that I should write a book. I was thinking about how much easier it would be for us if we could teach our customers how to better cooperate and communicate with their barber. I also started thinking about how our business has changed so much over the years. Many people don't even know what a barber *is* anymore. A lot of people have no idea that barbering and cosmetology are different schools, different skills, different businesses. Many people don't know the difference between a barber shop and a beauty salon. In the old days, there were clear differences between the two, but the times have changed. I get annoyed when I tell someone I'm a barber, and two minutes later, they refer to me as a hairdresser. I get annoyed when people refer to my barber shop as a salon.

It bothers me greatly that the skill of barbering is being phased out and the traditional barber seems to be going the way of the shoemaker. As one of the oldest professions in the world, it is a great business and a useful skill in our society. One of my aims with this book is to raise awareness and help to preserve the role of the traditional barber as a respected tradesman in our society. I feel that the public should be aware of the differences between barbers and cosmetologists. It is never my intention to sound like one is better than the other. Only that they are different. Each have their own field of expertise.

This book is also written to help the customer to increase their odds of getting the haircut and service they want and to have a more pleasant experience at the barber shop or salon. There are many ways customers actually *cause* the barber to cut their hair wrong or too short. The purpose of this book is to make the customer aware of the ways they often influence the barber to mess up their haircut. This book is designed to be entertaining as well as educational.

This book is my rant. It is my personal "Confessions" of the situations that make me become "Surly." It is about all the little things I always wanted to tell the customers, but was afraid I might offend them. At times it may seem that I dislike barbering and perhaps should find another way to make a living, but it is quite the opposite. I am very proud to be a barber and I love what I do! The hair business, whether barbering or cosmetology, is a very enjoyable vocation for the most part. We have a good time every day at work. Some days it seems bizarre to actually get paid for what I am doing. We make a good living, we work in an air-conditioned environment, we don't work long hours or overtime, and we get to meet and talk with people from all walks of life and of all ages. They have interesting life stories and issues going on in their daily lives. If we are looking for information on something, there is usually someone whom we can ask. There are days when the mechanic sitting in your chair tells you how to fix that funny knock in your car, or the computer man tells you how to fix the virus on your computer, or an interesting elderly man tells you about his life in the old days.

Recently, my air-conditioning system broke in the middle of a hot summer day. It just so happened that a man getting his hair cut was an a/c tech and offered to look at it for me right then. He fixed it within an hour for the fee of a free haircut. If I had to close the shop because of the heat and wait for a company to show up, it would have cost me not only the charge of the repair, but also the time in lost wages.

As with any occupation, barbering can be difficult as well as rewarding. It can be challenging on many levels. There are always those days when you wake up late, get stuck in traffic, and arrive to a shop full of uncooperative people and wind up your day feeling tired and irritated. There are many things customers do that can really make our day rough, even though most of them don't intend to. I think most people want to be pleasant, and to know what they can do to help.

This book is also designed to help barbers to make their customers aware of certain things so that they can enjoy their work more and go home happy instead of being physically and mentally worn out, due to dealing with the way customers make our job harder than it needs to be.

Some of my colleagues have expressed to me that customers might become nervous about behaving a certain way in the barber chair after reading this book. I sincerely hope that is not the case and it is certainly not my intention. I only wish to increase the customer's odds of being happy with the service provided.

I hope that I haven't scared anyone away from pursuing a career in barbering or hairstyling. On the contrary, I hope I may have influenced a reader into considering barbering as their vocation.

My main purpose with this book is to educate and facilitate a line of communication and mutual respect between the customer and the barber/stylist.

Many of the situations relate to both barbers and hairdressers, however some are specific only to barbers. Often, it's just easier to just say "barber" as opposed to "barber/hairstylist/beautician/hairdresser/cosmetologist" etc. There are too many terms to refer to a person who cuts hair. When writing on the history and the laws of barbering, I only know American barber history and laws, and I didn't take the time and energy to research the history and laws of barbering in other countries. This book is not intended to be a historical textbook or a legal guideline.

The History Of Barbers

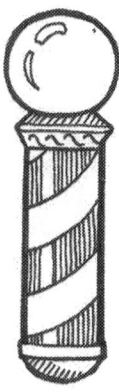

Today

One of the first things we learn in barber school is the history of barbering. It is a subject that I feel very passionate about, and is one the many reasons I am writing this book. Many people today are unaware that barbers were once surgeons and dentists and clergymen. The traditional barber pole is a symbol that comes from the bloody bandages blowing in the wind. The technical term for a barber is a tonsorial artist. When I was writing this book, I felt it would be important to include a chapter on the complete history of barbering because the book was inspired so greatly by the changes going on in the hair industry today. Barbering is becoming a lost art. When a man (or a woman) wants to become a barber today, they have to learn all of the cosmetology services in addition to barbering. They have to learn how to do permanent waves, hair-coloring, and putting rollers in people's hair. There are fewer and fewer men going to barber school, partly for that reason. It's becoming harder and harder to find male barbers. Even today, there are customers who have been around since WWII that prefer to have a male barber. They remember the days when there were no women barbers. It has become very difficult to find barbers at all, whether male or female, when we need to hire someone. I have a traditional barber shop. Sometimes I don't get a single call when I place an ad for help wanted, in the newspaper. In the twenty-four years that I've been a barber, I've seen a lot of changes. I've worked with a lot of elderly barbers who were barbers when the Beatles came out and started the long hair trend on men. A lot of barbers put their tools away and found other ways to put food on their tables rather than adapt to the changes. It was very hard on the barbers who did survive and learn the new tricks. Over the years, I've seen a lot more women becoming barbers and the barber schools now have more female than male students. Barbers used to be only men. There have been a lot of changes in recent years because of the unisex salons and people not knowing the difference between barbers and cosmetologists. In the old days, everyone knew what a barber was. These days, many people have no idea what a barber is.

I searched the internet for an article on the history of barbering and I found the following at http://www.barberpole.com. It's a really nice website and they kindly gave me permission to use this article.

Barbering Through The Ages

The word "barber" comes from the Latin word "barba," meaning beard. It may surprise you to know that the earliest records of barbers show that they were the **foremost men of their tribe.** They were the medicine men and the priests. But primitive man was very superstitious and the early tribes believed that both good and bad spirits, which entered the body through the hairs on the head, inhabited every individual. The bad spirits could only be driven out of the individual by cutting the hair, so various fashions of hair cutting were practiced by the different tribes and this made the barber the most important man in the community. In fact, the barbers in these tribal days arranged all marriages and baptized all children. They were the chief figures in the religious ceremonies. During these ceremonies, the hair was allowed to hang loosely over the shoulders so that the evil spirits could come out. After the dancing, the long hair was cut in the prevailing fashion by the barbers and combed back tightly so that the evil spirits could not get in or the good spirits get out.

In Egypt, many centuries before Christ, **barbers were prosperous and highly respected.** The ancient monuments and papyrus show that the Egyptians shaved their beards and their heads. The Egyptian priests even went so far as to shave the entire body every third day. At this time the barbers carried their tools in open-mouthed baskets and their razors were shaped like small hatchets and had curved handles. In Greece, barbers came into prominence as early as the fifth century, BC. These wise men of Athens rivaled each other in the excellence of their beards. Beard trimming became an art and barbers became leading citizens. Statesmen, poets and philosophers, who came to have their hair cut or their beards trimmed or curled and scented with costly essences, frequented their shops. And, incidentally, they came to discuss the news of the day, because the barber shops of ancient Greece were the headquarters for social, political, and sporting news.

In the third century, BC, the Macedonians under Alexander the Great began their conquest of Asia and lost several battles to the Persians who grabbed the Macedonians by their beards, pulled them to the ground and speared them. This resulted in a general order by Alexander that all soldiers be clean-shaven. The civilians followed the example of the soldiers and beards lost their vogue. Barbers were unknown in Rome until 296 BC, when Ticinius Mena came to Rome from

Sicily and introduced shaving. Shaving soon became the fashion and the barber shop became the gathering place for the Roman dandies. No people were better patrons of the barbers than the Romans. They often devoted several hours each day to tonsorial operations, which included shaving, hair cutting, hairdressing, massaging, manicuring and the application of rare ointments and cosmetics of unknown formulas. The great ladies of Rome always had a hairdresser among their slaves and the rich nobles had private tonsors, as they were then called. **Barbers were so highly prized that a statue was erected to the memory of the first barber of Rome.**

When Hadrian became emperor, beards became the fashion again and for a very good reason. Hadrian had a face covered with warts and scars. He allowed his beard to grow to cover these blemishes. The people of Rome imitated the emperor and grew beards whether they needed them or not.

The fashion changed again to clean-shaven faces. We know that Caesar was clean-shaven. As we will see repeated in history many times, the leaders of the state were the leaders of fashion and the people were always ready to follow the prevailing styles.

During the first centuries of the Christian era, the barbers of Europe practiced their profession wherever it was the custom to shave the face and trim the beard. Charlemagne made long, flowing hair the fashion, but each new conqueror changed the fashions according to his whim and personal needs. During the first ten centuries after Christ, the great majority of the people and even the nobles were uneducated and could neither read nor write. The most learned people of the times were the monks and priests who became the physicians of the dark ages. There were no professional surgeons at that time. Most of the diseases, which are easily curable now, were fatal then.

"Bloodletting" was the popular method of curing all ills. The clergy who enlisted barbers as their assistants first performed this. This was the first step in the upward progress of the barber profession. Barbers continued to act as assistants to the physician-clergy, until the 12th century. At the council of Tours in 1163, the clergy were forbidden to draw blood or to act as physicians and surgeons on the grounds that it was sacrilegious for ministers of God to draw blood from the human body. The barbers took up the duties relinquished by the clergy and the **era of barber-surgeons began. The connection between** *barbery* **and** *surgery* **continued for more than six centuries** and the barber profession reached its pinnacle during this time.

Surgeons

The earliest known organization of barbers was formed in 1096 in France when William, archbishop of Rouen, prohibited the wearing of a beard. The barber-surgeon, or "chirurgeons," began to thrive all over Europe. They were the doctors of the times and the royalty as well as the common people came to the barbers to have their ills treated as well as for shaving and hair-cutting. The physicians proper were in continual conflict with the barber-surgeons. The barbers performed dentistry as well as surgery and this brought down on them the enmity of the dentists of the times. This caused a long strife, whose settlement required the interference of kings and councils. But the barbers retained the privilege of practicing dentistry and surgery for several centuries.

In the middle of the 13th century, the barber companies of Paris, known as the Brotherhoods of St. Cosmos and St. Domain, founded the first school ever known for the systematic instruction of barbers in the practice of surgery. This school was later enlarged and became the model for schools of surgery during the Middle Ages. Many of the foremost surgeons of the times were students of the School of St. Cosmos and St. Domain. **The establishment of this school was one of the greatest contributions ever made toward the progress of humanity.** The oldest barber organization in the world, still known in London as the "Worshipful Company of Barbers," was established in 1308. Richard le Barbour, as the Master of the Barbers, was given supervision over the whole of his trade in London. Once a month he had to go the rounds and rebuke any barbers whom he found acting disgracefully or entering on other trades less reputable. The master of a city company not only had this power, but he successfully prevented unauthorized persons from practicing the barber profession. The Barbers Guild of the 14th Century was undoubtedly more powerful than any of the modern unions. The king and council sanctioned the Guilds and so they could enforce their regulations. It was not uncommon for violators of Guild regulations to suffer prison terms for their misdemeanors.

Up to the year 1416, the barbers were not interfered with in the practice of surgery and dentistry. But it was soon evident that they were attempting too much. It was impossible to expect ordinary human beings to competently practice surgery, dentistry and the various tonsorial operations. People began to complain that the barber-surgeons were making them sick instead of well. Many barber-surgeons resorted to quackery in order to cover up their ignorance of medicine and anatomy. These abuses came to the attention of the mayor and council of London. In 1416 an ordinance was passed forbidding barbers from taking under their care any sick person in danger of death or maiming, unless within three days after being called in, they presented the patient to one of the masters of the Barber-Surgeon's Guild. **Until 1461 the barbers were the only persons practicing surgery.** The practice of surgery was still in its primitive stage, but new discoveries were being made regularly and the barbers found it impossible to keep up with the new discoveries and at the same time maintain their skill in dentistry and barbering. The surgeons began to forge to the front and became increasingly jealous of the privileges accorded the barbers. But for a long time they could do nothing to prevent the barbers from acting as surgeons. In 1450, the Guild of Surgeons was incorporated with the Barbers Company by act of parliament. Barbers were restricted to bloodletting, toothdrawing, cauterization and the tonsorial operations. However the board of governors, regulating the operations of the surgeons and barber-surgeons, consisted of two surgeons and two barbers. Every time a surgeon was given a diploma entitling him to practice his profession, the diploma had to be signed by two barbers as well as two surgeons. The surgeons resented.this, but the barbers were very much favored by the monarchs and preserved their privileges until the middle of the 18th century. Henry VIII, Charles II and Queen Anne presented the barber-surgeons with valuable gifts and raised many of them to high offices. Under a clause in the Act of Henry VIII, the Barber-Surgeons were entitled to receive the bodies of four criminals each year who had been executed. The dissections were performed four times a year in the Barber-Surgeons Hall which still stands in London.

The modern barber pole originated in the days when bloodletting was one of the principal duties of the barber. The two spiral ribbons painted around the pole represent the two long bandages, one twisted around the arm before bleeding and the other used to bind is afterward. Originally, when not in use, the pole with a bandage wound around it, so that both might be together when needed, **was hung at the door as a sign**. But later, for convenience, instead of hanging out the original pole, another one was painted in imitation of it and given a permanent place on the outside of the shop. *This was the beginning of the modern barber pole.*

As the science of medicine, surgery and dentistry advanced, the barbers became less and less capable of performing the triple functions of barber-surgeon-dentist. The surgeons wished to be separated entirely from the barbers and they petitioned parliament to sever the ancient relationship of the barbers and surgeons and compel each profession to adhere strictly to its own provinces. A committee was appointed by parliament to investigate the matter and the petition was favorably reported to parliament. By an act of parliament, which received the sanction of the king, the alliance between the barbers and surgeons was dissolved in June, 1745. Two separate companies were formed and the property, formerly owned by the barbers and surgeons jointly, was divided among the two companies.

Profession Declines

This marked the decline of the barber profession. Similar action was taken in France under the reign of Louis XIV. Toward the end of the 18th century the barbers of Europe had completely relinquished their right to perform any of the operations of surgery and dentistry, except in the small towns and out-of-the-way places where doctors and dentists were not obtainable. After the barbers were prohibited from practicing medicine, surgery and dentistry, they **became mere mechanics and servants**, subject to the whims of fashion. When wigs became the fashion during the 18th and part of the 19th century, barbers became wigmakers. Their profession had lost its ancient dignity and barbers had **become laborers**, instead of professional men. In England, America and all over the civilized world, the **decline of the barber was a spectacle for all to see.** Barber shops became hangouts, places where low characters assembled. Smutty stories, malicious scandal and gossip of all kinds characterized barber shops until a few years ago. **A barber shop was a place where men showed their lower instincts and where women dared not enter.**

Late in the nineteenth century there were several noteworthy events in the barber profession that gave it an upward trend, and the effects are still carrying onward and upward. How long it will be before the barber may be looked up to as a professional man, taking his place by the side of the dentist, chiropodist, chiropractor and other kindred professions, cannot be foretold, but it would seem both the public and the profession are ready for better things. **In 1893, A. B. Moler of Chicago, established a school for barbers.** This was the first institution of its kind in the world, and its success was apparent from its very start. It stood for higher education in the ranks, and the parent school was rapidly followed by branches in nearly every principle city of the United States. In the beginning of schools, simply the practical work of shaving, haircutting, facial treatments, etc., was taught as neither the public nor the profession were ready to accept scientific treatments of hair, skin and scalp. Not until about 1920 was much effort made to professionalize the work.

The Business Of Barbering

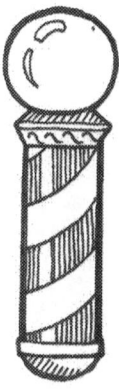

The Difference Between
Barbers And Cosmetologists

Over the years, the barber profession has evolved and changed to suit the public. In the past, barbers were men who shaved and cut men's hair. Hairdressers were women who cut women's hair and fixed it pretty. In a nutshell, barbers were and are still, primarily for men's grooming needs, and hairdressers were and are still, primarily for women's grooming needs. In the past, women were not allowed in the barber shop. It was unheard of. It was a place where men went to talk "guy talk" like politics, war, economy, etc., that women weren't privy to in those days. Some barber shops had spittoons lined up against the wall where the customers would spit while getting their hair cut. Before the disposable razor was invented, men had their own shaving mug with their name on it, and went to the barber shop to be shaved and groomed. Going to the barber shop was like reading the newspaper. It's where the men got the latest news. Some time during and after World War II, there became a need for women to get jobs and go to work outside the home and it became acceptable for women to practice barbering. In the past, a barber was hired as an apprentice and later became a barber after proving their skills. Presently, there are two different types of schools to learn the art of hair-cutting. There is Barber School. And there is Cosmetology School. They are different yet similar in many ways. They are two different licenses. There is a license to practice Barbering. And there is a license to practice Cosmetology. They are run and regulated by different laws in each state. There are Barber Schools and Barber Shops which are regulated and inspected by the Barber Board, which is a branch of the Department of Business and Professional Regulations, also known as the DBPR. Then there are Cosmetology Schools and Beauty Salons which are run by the Cosmetology Board, also a branch of the Department of Business and Professional Regulations. In the USA, each state has different regulations and laws.

In most states, barbers are allowed to work in beauty salons, and cosmetologists are allowed to work in barber shops. Some states still have an apprentice license, a barber license, and a master barber license. A student has to attend a certain number of hours in school, in order to apply to take the state board exam and acquire a license. We have to apply for a license for each state we live in and submit proof of the hours previously attended. Some states have stricter laws than others. In some states, we have to take another state board exam and/or attend more hours of school. We also have to renew our license every two years. Cosmetologists are sometimes required to attend a certain amount of continuing education, such as hair shows, classes and seminars between license renewals. Both barbers and cosmetologists have to submit proof of attending a course on the HIV virus. In some states, the owner must have a barber's license in order to display a barber pole as a sign, or to use the word "Barber" in the name of the shop.

Barbers generally don't shampoo the hair or fix it pretty. Most traditional barbers don't do permanent waves, hair coloring, curl sets, blow-drying or using the curling iron, although it is taught in the barber schools today. Barbers are trained primarily in the art of hair-cutting.

There are always exceptions to a rule. When I explain the differences between cosmetologists and barbers, I mean for it to taken in the "typical" or "most common" sense. There are barbers who can do beautiful style haircuts. There are barbers who can use a curling iron and a blow-dryer as good as any hairstylist can. There are cosmetologists who can do a beautifully tapered man's haircut as good as any barber. I'm sure there are cosmetologists who can shave with a straight razor too. Some have been taught by co-workers. Some have learned from practice and trial and error. But the main difference between the two is the man's military style, tapered haircut and the use of the straight razor. I do not mean to sound like I am insulting the cosmetologists. I'm only trying to define their field of expertise and the barber's field of expertise. If they both learn all of the same things, why are there two different schools, licenses, and laws?

Both barbers and cosmetologists are taught basic layered haircuts which are usually cut wet, holding the sections of hair with our fingers and cutting it with scissors. Barbers sometimes refer to layer cuts as "scissor cuts" or "style cuts" or "wet cuts." Cosmetologists are taught always holding the hair with their fingers. A basic layer cut that falls to the middle of a person's ear, is cut to the same length all over the head. (Ill. #1) A traditional man's haircut, called a "man's regular haircut," is cut above the ears and tapered in the back, military style, with the clippers and the comb, or scissors over the comb. A "taper" is when the hair on the neckline is cut on the skin with the clippers—0" length and gradually gets longer, eventually connecting to the length on top. (Ill. #2) A tapered hairline sort of looks like it just fades right into nothing. There is no distinct, blunt line on a taper. It's a very precise skill to master. If the barber stops too quick with the clippers, it will cut a "notch" in it. It's very difficult to cut the hair with the clippers right on the neck, and no comb under them. The barber has to rock the clippers out in just such a way to skillfully taper a hairline. It is *this* particular hair-cutting technique that makes the barber different. Cosmetologists are not taught the clipper over comb, (Ill. # 3) or scissor over comb (tapering) technique. (Ill. #4)

Illustration # 1 Basic Layer cut

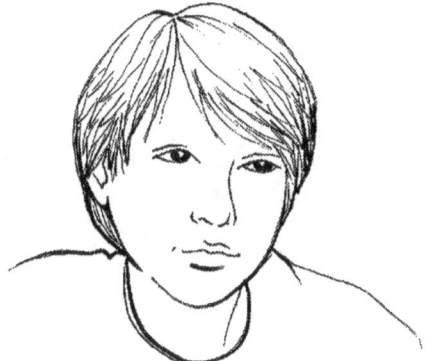

Illustration # 2 Tapered Hairline

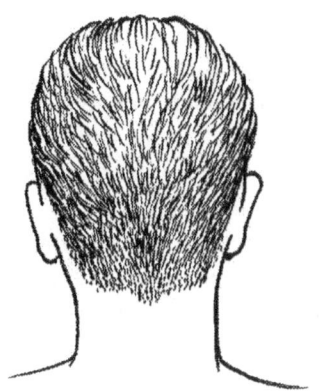

Illustration # 3 Clippers Over Comb

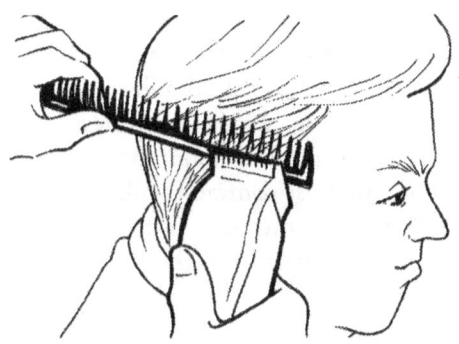

Illustration # 4 Scissors Over Comb

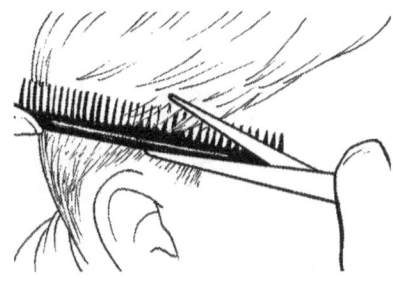

Regular men's haircuts are usually cut dry because the clippers are not designed for cutting wet hair, and the barber needs to see the blend. Men's military style, tapered haircuts are not the average cosmetologist's field of expertise, just as coloring or "setting" the hair isn't the average barber's field of expertise.

Barbers' tools are different than cosmetologists' tools. Most of a barber's tools are designed for cutting dry hair. We typically have three different clippers that we use. One is a large clipper that has interchangeable blades of different sizes. I'm sure there are several brands, but the most popular, or the "industry standard" is the Oster® #76 clipper. (Ill. #5) Oster® is the brand name. They make many clippers and other tools and gadgets including household toasters and blenders. The interchangeable blades are standard sizes that all Oster® clippers use. They are not guards that go over the blade to change the size. Most traditional barbers don't like to use those. They are designed for more light work. They're more suitable for hairdressers who don't use them as much as a barber does. For the amount of clipper work a hairdresser does, it doesn't pay to have an Oster® clipper, since they are much more expensive to purchase and you need to own all the different blades for them. The blades themselves cost $25.00 to $30.00 each. A barber needs a tough clipper that can be used all day long without getting too hot. The clipper that is used with the plastic guard gets very hot after about ten minutes of use. The plastic guards miss a lot of the hair, and can't hold up to the work barbers put the Oster® clipper through. We use the Oster® clippers for buzz cuts, burrs, bald cuts, princetons, wiffles, flat tops, crew cuts, fades, military haircuts, and beard trims. Some barbers use the Oster® clipper for tapering (clipper over comb) also, but it is not common.

Barbers usually have an all around basic clipper that has an adjustable blade that cuts from a size #000 (closed) to #1 (open)on the Wahl® or #1-1/2 (open) on the Andis Master® which are used most often in combination with a comb. The Wahl® and Andis.® brands seem to be the most common. (Ill. #6) These are the clippers that you attach the plastic guards onto, or use by themselves directly on the skin, or use with a comb. Most barbers hold the hair with the comb and cut it with the clipper with no guard. We use the basic clippers (with no guard) for tapering the hairline and going around the ears, and for close haircuts. We use these clippers on just about every man's haircut, unless it's a "layer" "style" "scissor" type of haircut.

We also use a small clipper called an "edger" or "T-edger" that cuts very close, much like an electric shaver. (Ill. #7) It is used for shaving the neck, making it clean cut around the ears, cutting the hair inside and on the ears, and some barbers use them to trim the eyebrows, nose hairs, and mustaches. If a man wants his head shaved completely bald or wants a beard shaved completely off, we can use the T-edger or we can also use the Oster® clipper with a #00000 blade which is the same. Or we can also use the standard clipper with the blade closed. The T-edger clipper is most commonly used as a finishing tool.

Illustration # 5A Oster® clipper   **Illustration # 5B Oster® blade**

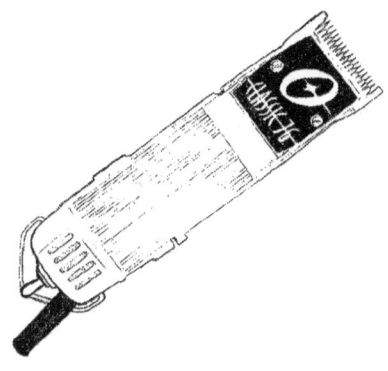
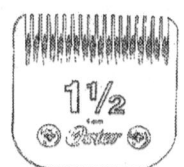

Illustration # 6A Andis®   **# 6B Wahl® clipper**   **# 6C plastic guard**

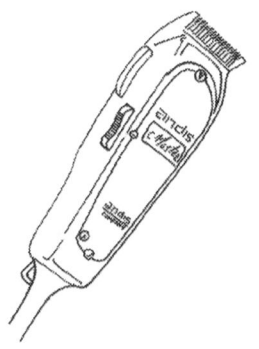
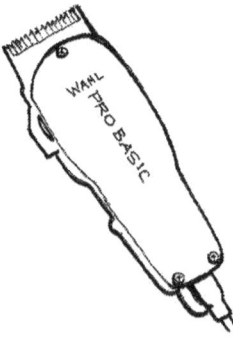
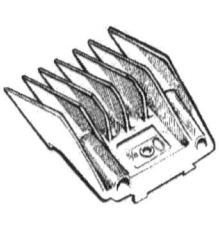

Illustration # 7 Edger

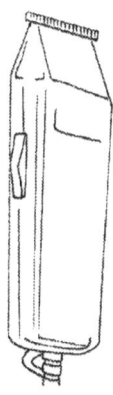

Barbers' scissors are called "shears." They are traditionally much larger than a hairdresser's shears and are used in a completely different fashion or technique. These shears are for blending the taper with the rest of the hair and gradually getting longer toward the top of the head. We hold the hair with the comb and cut with the shears which is called the "scissor over comb" technique. Sometimes the barber has smaller shears that we use on wet hair and layer cuts, or when we hold the hair in our fingers such as when we're cutting the top or layering the hair. Some barbers also use shears called "blending shears" sometimes referred to as "thinning shears." (**Ill. #8**) There is a difference between the two in the amount of teeth they have. Blending shears can be used as thinning shears, but thinning shears can't always be used as blending shears. It really depends on the barber and the technique they are using. When used as blending shears, they're used in the scissors over comb technique, and operated by cutting the hair many times in the same spot. When used as thinning shears, the hair is held up with either fingers or a comb, and cut one time approximately halfway from ends to root. It is not recommended to cut more than one time or to use them close to the root as they will create lots of short hairs that will stick straight up.

Illustration # 8 Thinning Shears

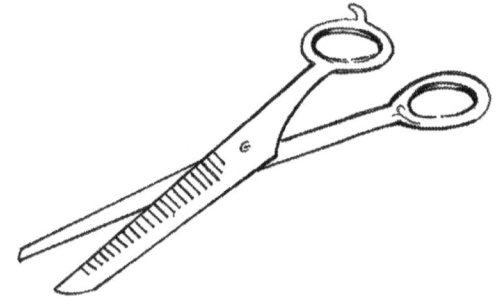

We also use several different types of combs. We use a wide comb, called a "flat top comb" that is used for flat tops and for cutting major bulk with the clippers. We have "styling combs" which are a basic firm plastic comb, that we use for most of the work. Then we have a "taper comb" which is a light, flexible plastic that tapers to a smaller size on one end, that we use for tapering and really close to the skin hair-cutting. Different barbers prefer different combs. There are too many combs and too many preferences to list them all. There is no standard preference.

When a hairdresser cuts a man's hair that is too short to hold with their fingers, (for instance, the hair around the ears and on the nape of the neck might only be 1/16" long) they usually will put a plastic guard over their clippers and cut the sides and back that way, then blend it in to the rest of haircut. If they do a fade or buzz cut, they use a plastic guard on their clipper also. The guards come in many sizes, but they do not correspond to an Oster® clipper's blades. This causes some confusion, which we'll discuss in a later chapter.

Hairstylists' shears (scissors) are commonly smaller, and more expensive than a barber's. Because they usually shampoo their customer's hair first, they are designed primarily for cutting wet, clean hair. Cosmetologists use tools such as blow-dryers, curling irons, and brushes of all different sizes and shapes. They also use rollers, hairpins, teasing combs and all sorts of styling products.

Barbers usually don't work by appointments, although there are exceptions. Most barbers shops are run on a walk-in basis. Typical time for a man's regular haircut is approximately fifteen minutes for most barbers. Some are faster. Some are slower. A barber's job is hair-cutting. Most barbers can do all types of haircuts and charge accordingly. Some barbers only do traditional haircuts and don't want to do anything else. Many senior barbers only know traditional men's haircuts. In my experience, barbers most commonly cut the customer's hair facing away from the mirror and counter for several reasons. The electric cords from our clippers need to reach without stretching across the customer or hanging in their face. Barbers also use the mirror to look at the blend on a taper haircut. We can see mistakes such as lines, holes, notches and steps better in the mirror.

Hairdressers typically cut and fix ladies' hair. They fix the hair pretty. They put it in rollers, blow-dry it, use curling irons, tease the hair, do permanent waves and hair coloring. They usually use a variety of products such as styling gel, mousse, and hair sprays. Most salons these days also offer manicures, pedicures, waxing, facials, massage therapy and many other services. Hairdressers most commonly work by appointments because they spend variable amounts of time with their customers.

At some point in time, men started going to hairdressers and women started going to barber shops. The inception of "unisex salons" has changed the business drastically. The public is often unaware that there is even a difference between barbers and cosmetologists these days. There is a great deal of difference in the way we work, our techniques, laws, licenses, the tools we prefer to use and the services we prefer to do.

In my opinion, if you are a woman, (or a man with long hair), who likes their hair to be shampooed, cut, and styled, or if you want more than *just* a haircut (such as a perm/color etc) you should go to a salon/hairdresser. If you are a man (or a woman with short hair), and you don't care about getting (and paying for) a shampoo and having the hair fixed pretty afterward, you should go to a barber. Young boys should go to a barber. With young girls, it would really just depend on what you want done to their hair and how much money you want to spend. If a young girl is just getting a trim or a simple haircut, a barber shop is fine. If she has long hair, she should go to a stylist as it would be time consuming for a barber. If you are looking for a basic haircut, with a minimal loss of time, whether male or female, a barber shop is probably right for you. If you are looking for someone to fuss over you, and take some time on you, or if you get a fancy haircut, or you have extraordinarily thick or long hair, I recommend going to a salon where they have a receptionist and schedule appointments. In a walk-in situation, which is typical of barber shops, the barbers only have so much time to work on a haircut, because there are other haircuts waiting in line, and no one wants to wait long.

Most of the cosmetologists I've known love styling the hair and coloring it, and making it fabulous. Most have little or no interest in cutting hair except as a means to an end. Cutting men's hair is not usually what they want to do in a salon like that. And visa versa, barbers have little or no interest in styling and fixing the hair. Most barbers like to keep things simple and uncomplicated. Typically, barbering is much less egocentric. In the traditional barber shops that I've worked in, there always seems to be one "showy" barber. The other barbers will usually tease the "showboat" barbers. In beauty salons, they tend to praise each other's work, and "show off" the great work they do.

In the medical field, you have heart doctors, lung doctors, foot doctors etc. They have all gone to medical school and they are all in the field of medicine, but their training and their experience is different. You wouldn't go to a lung doctor for heart surgery, or a foot doctor for brain surgery, but they are all doctors of medicine. Just like you wouldn't take a car with brake problems to a transmission center. Yes, they are both mechanics, but they have a different field of expertise. It's the same kind of thing in the hair business. Barbers and Cosmetologists are both in the hair business, but they have two completely different fields of expertise. In all of my personal experience, I have never known a barber or a cosmetologist who feels that we compete with each other. There really is no intended competition between barber shops and beauty salons. I've worked in several barber shops in shopping centers with a salon right next door. In some cases we even refer customers to each other.

There are 3 common methods to manage barber shops and beauty salons: There are appointment shops, walk-in shops, and sign-in shops. There are many ways the customer can contribute and cooperate in each system so that the system runs smoothly. Very few people in our society have extra time to waste. No one likes to wait in line. Everyone has other things they would rather be doing. Children would rather be out playing with other children or watching cartoons. Working people and parents always have a serious time shortage. Even retired people have things they would rather be doing.

Each system is designed to save everyone involved as much time as possible, to lessen the amount of wait time, and to give each customer their fair amount of time in the chair. One system might work well for some people, while another system might work better for others. Each system is fair when all the parts of the system are working correctly. All the parts of the system work together. When one part of the system fails, it messes everyone up. There are many things that can go wrong.

Walk—In Shops

In a walk-in shop (typical of most barber shops) customers are taken in the order they come in the door. The barbers take turns taking customers when business is slow. When all the chairs are busy, whichever barber finishes the customer they are working on, takes the next customer in line. Some haircuts take longer than others. Some barbers are faster than others. Some barbers are more skilled or more experienced, and are able to do a better haircut than others. Customers sometimes wait for their favorite barber. That's fine if they want to wait. This should not hurt the other barbers' feelings. Each barber has people who wait for them. The more years a barber works in the same shop, the more customers will be waiting for them, and the more money they will make. They build what we call a following or a clientele of customers. A good barber will build their following in less time because people like their haircuts. The barbers build their own chair up, and business for the shop increases, when customers return. The barbers who make the most money in a barber shop are the ones who stay the busiest. The more barbers there are, the more haircuts can be done at once. The more business a shop builds, and the busier it becomes, the more barbers are hired to work, thus making the owner more money.

The owner of the shop gets a percentage of the money and the barber gets a percentage of the money, plus their tips. Barber shops typically pay 70%-75% commission to the barber. For example: 70% of $12.00 = 8.40 + tip. 75% of $14.00 = $10.50 + tip. Sometimes barber shops work on a chair rental system. On a chair rental system, the barber pays the owner a set amount of money each day, no matter how many haircuts they do.

Barbers are usually self-employed. There are no benefits such as paid days off, paid vacations, health insurance, or retirement funds. Barbers usually pay their own taxes, which means paying double social security tax. (When an employer takes taxes out for an employee, the employer matches the SS tax.) If the owner of the shop pays a high commission, they will get barbers who are more experienced and have more skill. The customers will be pleased and will be more likely to refer others to the shop. Better barbers will build more clientele, thus making the owner, and the other barbers, more profit. The more barbers there are, the more haircuts can be done at the same time.

When you go to a walk-in shop, don't assume that all the people in the waiting area are there to get a haircut. Some of the people are just waiting for someone else who is getting a haircut. Often, an entire family will come along for one hair cut. A parent can't very well leave small children home alone when they take one of their children to get a haircut. Children have to have someone to drive them. Many elderly people have to have someone to drive them too. Some of the customers might be waiting for one particular barber. One of the barbers may have stepped out for a moment, leaving the shop temporarily short handed. Maybe they just ran to the bank to get change and will be back quickly. Perhaps one is out for lunch and will be returning soon. If you have a limited amount of time, ask one of the barbers, usually the one in the front chair, how long the wait will be. It's impossible to give an accurate, precise waiting time, but he/she can usually give you a "ballpark estimate" based on the number of barbers working and the number of customers waiting.

There is usually one barber, (usually in the front chair) possibly the owner or manager who should know what's going on. It's tough for the barbers to know what's going on in the waiting room, and also pay attention to the customer in their chair at the same time, but someone has to do it. Number systems like the ticket machine in deli's work poorly for barber shops. The barber in the front chair still has to stop and remind each customer to get a ticket, or else one will inevitably forget, and then become upset when he realizes he's been skipped. Generally the owner or manager, or whoever is in the front chair is in charge of greeting the customers and paying attention to who is waiting for which barbers, and what barbers are leaving and when etc. It's not an easy job to do. Sometimes he has to stop in the middle of the haircut he is doing so he can think about it and calculate a wait time. If the average time for the barber is fifteen minutes per haircut, and there are four barbers working, two of which are almost finished, and two of which just got started, the first customer in line will be in the chair shortly, as will the next customer. (because two of the barbers are almost finished.) The third and fourth in line will have a ten to a fifteen minute wait. The fifth customer in line will be waiting fifteen to twenty minutes, assuming the first barber to finish got the first customer waiting and will be finished in fifteen minutes. If the shop has ten barbers, the first ten customers in line will be waiting five to fifteen minutes. The eleventh customer will have to wait fifteen to thirty minutes. If the shop has only one barber and there is no one ahead of you, figure on waiting five to fifteen minutes. If there is one person ahead of you, figure on waiting fifteen to thirty minutes. Five to ten minutes to finish the one in the chair plus ten to fifteen minutes to finish the one ahead of you who's waiting.

Once you have decided to sit down and wait, make sure to be aware of who is ahead of you in line, and who came in after you. The barber in the front chair is trying to help, but he has to pay attention to the haircut he's working on too. The customer in his chair will get nervous if he doesn't appear to be paying attention to what he is doing. It is best if the customer knows where they are in line. Most barbers can't handle cutting hair and directing traffic at the same time. Some shops don't have a barber who does this, or the boss/manager/first chair barber may not be there at all times.

When you know you're going to be next in the chair, *please wait until the barber calls for you*. The barber needs to give their full attention to the customer in their chair until the job is completely finished which includes taking their money and saying goodbye. Please allow the barber time to clean the hair off the chair, clean his tools and hold on to the chair, before you come over. There are safety issues when a customer gets in the chair without waiting for the barber to be there behind it. The chairs spin and are sometimes dangerous. There are also sanitation issues. I like to use the analogy of someone sitting down at a dirty table in a restaurant. Why would someone want to sit in the chair before it's been cleaned off?

When the shop is extremely busy, it becomes difficult for the barbers to stop long enough to get away for lunch. They may have to just stop and declare to the shop at large that they are going to lunch and will be unable to take the next person. While that may be irritating to a customer who has been waiting and is up next, I don't feel that a hungry barber is the best chance of a good haircut. Hunger often causes a person's hands to shake and usually makes a person irritable. Expect a fast, sloppy haircut if you sit in a hungry barber's chair! I would not want to have an irritable barber with shaking hands cutting my hair! Chances are good that the barber has timed it to where one of the others will be finished in the next few minutes.

If you have a favorite barber you like to wait on, it would be courteous to ask the barber if it's ok to wait for them and if they've had lunch yet, or if they are going anywhere soon. The barber may have others in front of you and/or may have somewhere they need to go. Perhaps they have a lunch date with their child, or a dentist appointment, or something of that nature. A barber who has a large following has a difficult time coordinating a break for anything in a busy walk-in shop. Obviously, it's best for the customer if the shop has several good barbers they can go to. Customers don't like to wait. However, barbers do like to make money! If a shop has too many barbers and not enough customers coming in, the barbers don't make as much money. It's a long day sitting around staring at each other. There is nothing to do if there isn't a customer to work on. If there are too many customers and not enough barbers, the customers tend to get impatient and may leave to go someplace else.

In a walk-in shop, you would have to have a crystal ball to know how many barbers you need each day. There is absolutely no way to know when it will be busy and when it will be slow except on an "average" basis. If the shop is closed on Mondays, chances are good that it will be busy on Tuesdays. If it's a retirement community, chances are good it will be busier in the mornings, and quiet at lunch time. If there is a local lady's golf day, (the men can't play golf) chances are good it will be busy on that day. In a metropolitan area, (working men) chances are good it will be busy at lunch time and late in the afternoons. Saturdays are usually busy in all shops. Entire families with two or three haircuts come in all at one time, making it busy instantly. Saturdays are the only option for many children with working parents. Barber shops are always a little short-handed during the lunch hours, (11:30 AM-2:00 PM) because they ordinarily take turns going to lunch, leaving the shop short-handed for a while, unless they close the shop up for lunch and all eat at the same time. The week before major holidays such as Easter, Christmas, and New Year's Eve are typically busy. The week before school starts is very busy with children. The week of school pictures is often very busy with children. The barber shop can't very well hire extra barbers for those weeks and then fire them all the next day, so customers should be prepared to have a longer wait time or not come during those busy times.

Walk-in type barber shops *typically* don't wash, blow-dry, or "set" the hair. It's ok if your hair is not perfectly clean, or is messed up. It's not pleasant if you come in with it extremely dirty. It's best not to have a lot of gel, hair-spray, or other sticky products in the hair. I recommend to arrive with your hair dry. Barbers generally cut the hair dry, with clippers over comb, or scissors over comb, or wet it with a squirt bottle and leave it wet. We must be able to see if everything is blending, which is difficult when the hair is wet. Clippers are not designed to cut wet hair. Some (most) barbers prefer to do the clipper work and the blending work while the hair is dry, then wet it and cut the top holding the hair with our fingers.

Barbers in walk-in shops increase their income only by doing more haircuts or raising the price of haircuts. The haircut prices in a walk-in type barber shop do not vary in large degrees because they only do services that take an average of fifteen to twenty minutes to do. Some charge a flat rate for all haircuts. Some charge one price for men and one price for ladies. Some offer a discount to children and/or senior citizens. Some have a price for "regular haircuts" (clippers) and a price for "style" (scissors) haircuts. Some have a price for short haircuts and go up according to the length of the hair. The prices are based on the average amount of time it takes. There is no way to make all the people happy all the time. Sometimes ladies get mad because they have to pay more. It takes longer to do a lady's layer cut than it does for a man's clipper cut. If a lady wants her hair cut very short with the clippers like a man's, then the shop may make an exception. Most barber shops will cut mustaches, eyebrows, and ear and nose hairs, for no extra charge, as part of the haircut.

The neck is always shaved in a barber shop unless the customer requests not to. Some barber shops still shave the neck and around the ears with hot lather and a straight razor, but because of HIV and economical issues, most shops shave the neck with electric trimmers nowadays. Beard trims are very time consuming, so they will typically cost only a few dollars less than a haircut. Most shops will trim a little girl's bangs for a small fee, such as $3.00 to $5.00.

Customers seldom enjoy waiting, so speed is important in a walk-in shop. A busy walk-in type barber shop cannot spend fifteen minutes discussing how you want your hair cut. If you require consultation, or if you want someone to spend a long time with you, you might want to consider one of the other options such as making an appointment at a salon. I feel that an average of a ten minute wait is fair to both the barbers and the customers. Remember that more experienced barbers are going to work where they can make more money. If there is never a long wait, chances are good that the shop is overstaffed. They will then have a high turnover rate of barbers, and may not last long in business.

Just about everything in life requires a minimum of a ten minute wait. You wait more than ten minutes to see a doctor, a dentist, eye doctor, or chiropractor even when you have an appointment. Making a simple phone call these days requires at least ten minutes of time to get through all the menus and finally get to speak to a human being! Getting a haircut is relaxing. It feels good. It doesn't cost much money, and it keeps you looking good for several weeks. If you think about it, a haircut lasts the average person approximately one month. If you pay $12.00 for a haircut, and you divide that $12.00 by the thirty days in a month, it comes to .40 cents per day. I feel it is worth waiting ten minutes for a good quality haircut from a barber who is happy with their occupation, and with their present job, because they are making a decent living and their boss is fair to them by not overstaffing. If time is more important to you than having a happy, pleasant barber, then you might want to consider another option such as making an appointment.

Appointment Salons And Shops

Full service beauty salons are typically run by appointments. There is usually a receptionist who answers the phone and sets up the appointments for the hairstylists. This person's salary is derived from the shop's income, so you'll usually find the hair services to be more expensive to cover such costs. Establishments offering several types of services, as opposed to *just* haircuts, usually have to run by appointments because some services take longer than others such as the following:

short basic hair cut .... average time: 15 minutes
long thick hair cut .... average time: 30 minutes
shampoo and condition .... average time: 10 minutes
blow-dry/style .... average time: 15 minutes
shampoo/cut/style .... average time: 45 minutes
permanent wave .... average time: 2-4 hours
color treatment .... average time: 1-3 hours

The receptionist who schedules appointments finds out what services the customer wants, and sets it in a block of time needed for that particular hairstylist to do the service requested. On a perfect day, the customer arrives on time, the hairstylist is running on time, the service rendered comes out perfect and takes exactly the average amount of time to do. As the customer is checking out, the next customer walks in the door in the same moment and so forth throughout the day. But ... that's on a perfect day! There are so many things that can go wrong! Most often a perfect day starts going downhill when just one (all it takes is one) customer is late. Five minutes late isn't too bad. The stylist will just be slightly rushed, which isn't exactly to your favor. The stylist has no choice. If he/she can catch up on time it will prevent a dominoes effect whereas he/she becomes five minutes late on the next customer, then ten minutes late for the next one ... and so forth. If the customer is more than fifteen minutes late, they will likely have to reschedule the appointment, because there simply isn't sufficient time available. Seven to eight minutes late is a tough one to call. If they squeeze you in, expect to be rushed somewhat and try not to be overly particular. I suggest to apologize, try not to do it again, and tip the stylist generously.

There are many ways a stylist can get behind. The stylist could get an emergency phone call from their child's school and have to arrange a back up plan or get a babysitter. Time spent on the phone sets the hairstylist behind. Often, a service given takes longer than the time allotted on the book for them. If the stylist blocks 2 hours for a perm, and the client has longer or thicker than average hair, it will take more time, and will set the stylist behind. It's not the customer's fault, it's not the receptionist's fault, nor is it the hairstylist's fault. There is no blame to be placed on anyone, but it happens quite often, and the time has to be taken from somewhere else. Sometimes a service doesn't render the desired result and the time spent on extra modification wasn't planned for. For instance, a haircut isn't short enough and the customer wants it cut shorter. It will take the stylist another ten to fifteen minutes to re-cut it. A color service could come out too light or the wrong shade, and the stylist might have to correct it, but didn't allow for the extra time involved. Extra time is often taken up in the consulting/talking phase of the hair service. Full-service salons generally take into account a certain amount of time for consulting with the client to establish what they want done, but there is sometimes a misunderstanding or someone needs to explain something that is more complicated than expected.

These type of salons generally charge more than a walk-in type shop in order to pay for the receptionist's salary, for products used on the hair, and to pay rent on a much larger store space than a small shop, among other things. These type of salons usually pay their stylists anywhere from 50% to 65% commission. A large percentage of their income comes from tips. It's customary to tip a percentage of the charges, such as 15-20% however, a good stylist who goes the extra mile to make a customer happy will receive better tips. For example: 50% of a $12.00 haircut = $6.00 + tip. 65% of a $20.00 haircut or service = $13.00 + tip. The stylist earns more income by working in a more expensive salon, getting a higher commission, building a clientele, selling more expensive services to the customer, selling products to the customer, and receiving generous tips. Better skilled and more experienced stylists will want to work where the commission is high, business is good, prices are fair, and quality products are being supplied. In the more prestigious salons, benefits are often available. To get a raise in this business is to either raise the price of the services, raise the amount of commission paid, or build more business.

Sign—In Shops

There are more and more chain operated haircut shops opening up all over the country. They are most often a franchised operation. They are large corporations and are managed completely different than the "mom and pop" shops of yesteryear. There are many tiers of employment, and room for advancement. There is the low man on the totem pole—the hair-cutter. The owner of the shop can't be in every one of them, so a manager is needed to operate the shop. There are regional managers, supervisors, bookkeepers, payroll etc.

There are many salaries to be accounted for with the income produced. They have large staffs of hair-cutters and they are open longer hours than the average barber shop or beauty salon. These are really not barber shops or beauty salons, but are a sort of a merge between the two. They are typically a full-service salon in that they offer all types of hair services and sell products, but they focus primarily on inexpensive, quick haircuts. Employees can be hired using a barber's license, or a cosmetologist's license. Each person they hire goes through a training period to learn their method of hair-cutting and other services.

Most are cosmetologists just getting out of school, trying to gain experience. The haircut prices are low and the commissions paid to the hair-cutters are low. They are usually operated on a "sign-in" basis, whereas when a customer comes in, a person greets them and asks them to please sign in, and lets them know how long the wait is. Barber shops seldom operate on this system, because they would have to charge more money for the haircuts or pay the barbers less, in order to pay the person who makes sure everyone gets signed in. While in theory, if you post signs telling everyone to please sign in, everyone would see it and take care of themselves, it just doesn't work that way. Someone forgets to sign in, or someone leaves and comes back after his name has been called. Someone has to be in charge. That person has to be paid. That money has to come from somewhere. If the price of the haircut is low, then you can be assured it's coming from paying the hair-cutters a low commission.

Once a stylist gains experience and builds up some clientele, they tend to go find a better job somewhere, often taking their clientele with them, to a shop that charges more and pays a higher commission. 50% of a $12.00 haircut = $6.00 + $1.80 tip = $7.80. That is significantly less than 65% of a $18.00 haircut =

$11.70 + $2.70 tip = $14.40. It is common for this type of shop to include the shampoo in the base price, whether the customer wants it or not. Franchised shops often take taxes out for the employee, and pay in a weekly or bi-weekly paycheck. They open earlier and stay open later in the evenings than most salons and barber shops. They hire full-time and part-time employees. Because of the low pay scale and the long hours, they have a high turnover rate of hair-cutters, as they move on to find better jobs. Don't expect to see the same person who cut your hair the last time you were there. Hair-cutters who are good at what they do tend to work in higher paying shops or salons.

The Haircut Experience

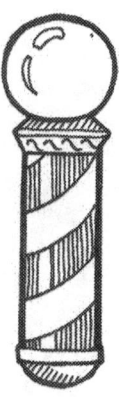

The Basic Principles Of Hair Cutting

The art of hair-cutting is built on the principle of geometry. Without going into the full details of how to cut hair, I will try to explain in simple terms what we do when we pick up the hair and cut it. We use our comb to divide the hair apart in sections. We take a-hold of the hair with our fingers, right behind the comb, and follow the comb with our fingers held tautly onto the hair, out to the length where we want to cut it. (**Ill. # 9**) We cut along our fingers in a straight line. Once we have started cutting somewhere on the head, we use that section as a "guide" and use that length, and the angle of our fingers, to connect all the hair together, section by section, to that length. It works sort of like a "dot to dot."

Illustration # 9 Holding hair with fingers

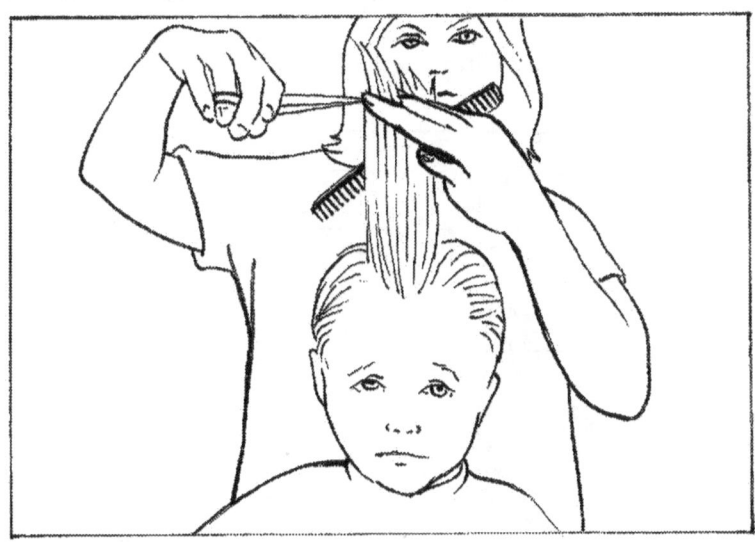

If we cut the hair on top 3" long and the length in the back is going to be 3" long, we connect the dots, section by section, angling our fingers toward our goal. (**Ill. # 10**)

Illustration #10 Basic Layer Cut (diagram)

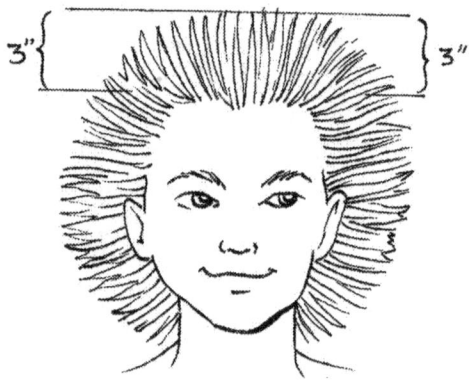

If we cut the hair on top 3" long and the length in the back is going to be 8" long, we connect the dots, section by section, angling our fingers toward our goal. (**Ill. # 11**)

Illustration # 11 Long Layer Cut (diagram)

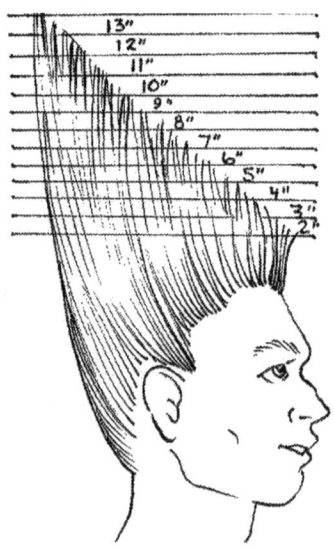

All the hair has to connect together with precision or it will be uneven.

On a man's tapered haircut, which is too short to hold with our fingers, we use the clippers against the skin, at first, then we use the comb to hold the hair. We start at the bottom and graduate the hair longer and longer as we go up the head. It's all about aim. The hair is held exactly where we want to cut it, and then we aim for it with the cutting instrument. It's very hard to do, actually. If we miss our aim with the cutting instrument, and cut a piece shorter than the rest, it will leave a "line" or "step" or "hole" in the cut. It's not as easy as it looks. Having been a barber for twenty-four years now, I still make mistakes sometimes. If the customer moves, or we miss our aim, cutting the surrounding hair shorter is the only way to fix it and blend it in. Most minor boo-boos can be fixed, but sometimes it leads to a shorter haircut than we intended. After we establish our length, we blend it all together, "cross-check," and then, "fine-tune" it. People tend to think we are still cutting the hair shorter and shorter when we start going back through it. When we're fine tuning it, we are just getting what we missed, blending, and checking our work to make sure everything is even. We're not necessarily cutting it shorter. It is called a precision haircut for a reason.

Types Of Haircuts

There are basic, traditional haircuts and there are fad haircuts. Most adult men and little boys wear traditional type haircuts. When kids reach a certain age, they want to start wearing the haircut everyone else is wearing at the time. Regular Hair Cuts, Flat Tops, Crew Cuts, Buzz Cuts, Princetons, Whiffles, High and Tights etc., are all traditional men and boys' haircuts.

Fad haircuts don't usually come out with a specific name. The barber usually knows what's popular at the time. The kids just have to be able to describe it a bit. There is a haircut that is popular with young boys in my area right now that is basically a short hair cut buzzed on the sides with the clippers, cut short on top and spiked up in the front only, with the crown area smooshed flat down on the head with styling gel. We call it the "flip in the front" haircut. I've heard it called a "ski-slope" too. Sometimes "spike" haircuts are popular which is where the hair on the top is cut very short, and combed back so that it sticks up on top. A couple of years ago, the "Mushroom" haircut was fashionable. It was buzzed on the sides and then the top was long and hung over the sides with a distinct line (like a mushroom) around the head. Before that, "Surfer Cuts" were popular. They were buzzed short on one side up to the side part, and then the other side was long and hung over the side with a distinct line.

Any haircut on a boy or man that is above the ears, above the collar, and blended in together is called a "Regular" Haircut. It can be a tapered (graduated) hairline in the back, or it can be "blocked" in the back, which is cut straight across and has a definite blunt bottom of the hairline. If you desire to wear your hair longer, or to cover part of the ear, that would be called a "Layer Cut" or a "Scissor cut." Layer cuts are usually cut wet, holding the hair with the fingers, and cutting it with the scissors.

Illustration # 12 Regular Haircut
(Tapered back)

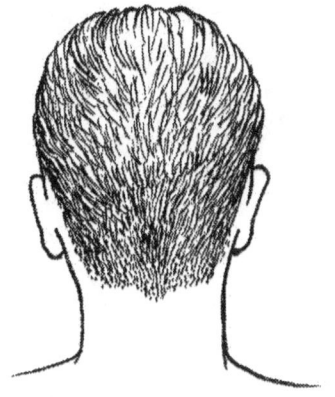

Illustration # 13 Regular Haircut
(Blocked back)

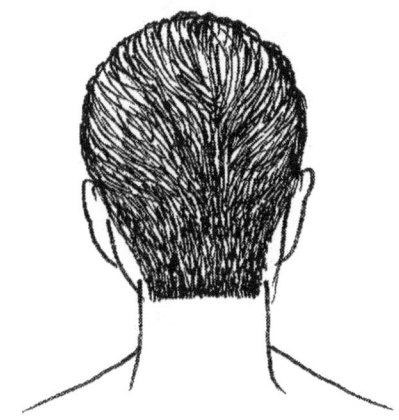

Illustration # 14 Buzz Cut

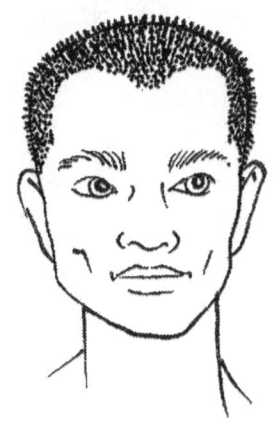

Illustration # 15 Flat—Top

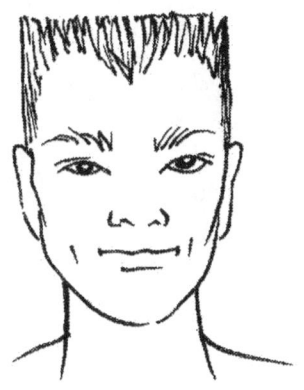

Illustration # 16 Mushroom

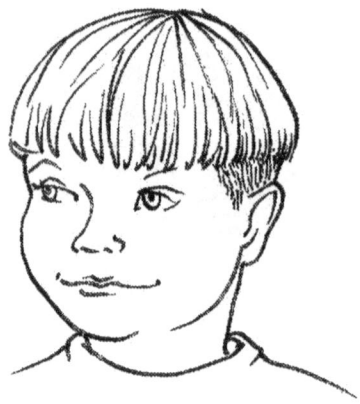

Illustration # 17 Flip In Front

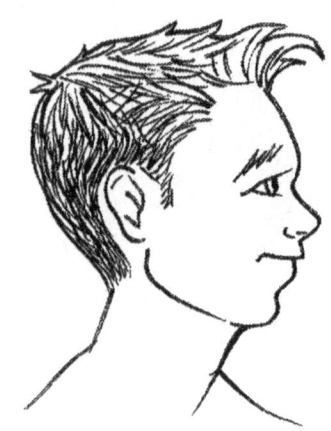

Illustration # 18 Fade

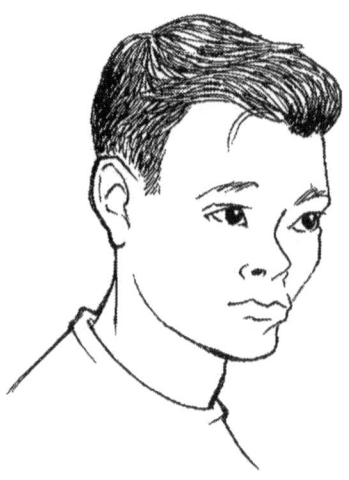

Illustration # 19 Skin fade

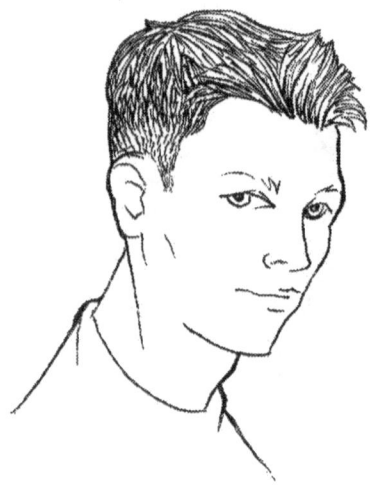

Illustration # 20 short layer cut　　**Illustration # 21 long layer cut**

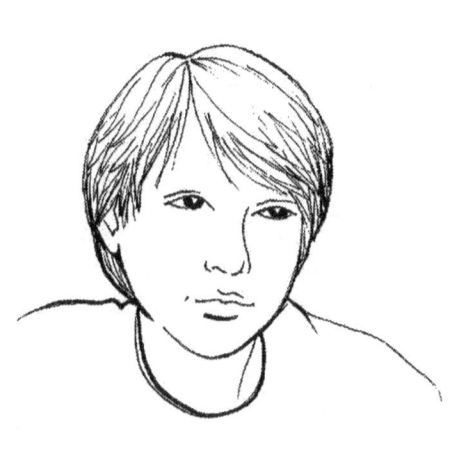 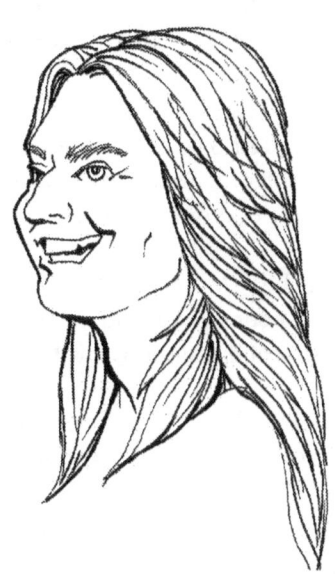

Names and types of hair-cuts:

BALD: A style in which all the hair on the scalp is removed with a razor. This is a popular haircut among athletes and men who are naturally balding.

BANGS: The section of hair that falls over the forehead. Can be worn down over the forehead, brushed to the side or brushed back.

BLOCKED NAPE: Blocking is when a visible line is created with the clippers at the nape. This is the most common type of finishing at the neck, but not always the most desirable. The disadvantage of a blocked hairline is that it does not grow out neatly and can make a thick neck look too wide.

BOWL HAIRCUT: This haircut was common in the depression era because it was an easy haircut to do at home. A bowl was placed on the head and all of the hair below was removed. Commonly called a "mushroom" cut today, it is popular among young teens and children.

BRUSH CUT: The sides and back are cut as for a crewcut. The top is cut the same length, about one-quarter to one-half inch over the top, following the contour of the head. The hair is then combed up so that the top resembles the bristles of a brush.

BURR: Hair over the entire head is cut one length, usually 1/8" or shorter. This is the type of haircut that new military recruits receive upon entering the service. This is a good option for someone who wants a no-maintenance haircut.

BUSINESS MAN'S CUT: Most popular among working professionals who require a conservative look. Normally, hair is cut with a slight taper on the sides and back and the top is left long enough to part and comb to the side.

BUTCH: This is a short version of the basic crewcut. Hair is left no longer than 1/4" on top and neatly tapered around the ears and at the back of the head.

BUZZCUT: A general term used to refer to haircuts that are done entirely with clippers. Technically speaking, there is no "official" style which can be called a buzzcut. See the following: butch, burr, brush cut, and crewcut, and whiffle.

CAESAR: A semi-short hairstyle made popular by Julius Caesar. The hair is layered to 1" to 3" on top and brushed forward with short bangs at the front. This cut is a low-maintenance style and is ideal for covering a receding hairline.

CLASSIC TAPER: Commonly referred to as a short business man's cut or graduation. The hair is left long enough to comb on top and gradually tapers down to 1/8 inch around the ears and the neck. This is a very traditional men's cut that is appropriate for any lifestyle.

CREW CUT: Also known as a short pomp or brush cut. The hair is cut short on the sides and back with the hair on top graduated in length from the front of the hairline to the back of the crown. The top hair, from side to side, should form a slight curve to conform to the general contour of the head.

FADE: The term "fade" originated in ethnic shops and has now become the popular term for an aggressively tight taper. Hair at the sides and back is cut as close as possible with clippers and "fades" or tapers up into almost any length on top. In some cases this haircut is mistakenly called a "military reg," which is misleading because each branch of the service has different regulations regarding hair length.

FAUX HAWK: This is a basic tapered haircut in which the hair is styled into a point at the center. It resembles a Mohawk, but without the shaved sides. The style can be worn as a Faux Hawk or styled differently for a conservative look.

FLAT TOP: The sides and back are cut similar to a crewcut, except the hair is cut on top with emphasis on flatness. The corners of the top are cut to give a square look. Variations include: "**Flattop with Fenders**," in which the hair on the sides is left longer and brushed back, giving the hair on the sides the appearance of fenders over the wheel of a car; also the "**Horseshoe**," which is an extremely short flattop. Viewed from the top, the hair resembles a horseshoe.

GRADUATION: Also referred to as a short business man's cut or classic taper. The hair is left long enough to comb on top and gradually tapers down very close around the ears and the neck. This is a very traditional men's cut that is appropriate for any lifestyle.

HIGH AND TIGHT: A very common haircut among US Marines, Army Rangers, and athletes. The hair is cut "high and tight" on the sides and back (zero length up to the crown). The top is usually crewcut length. The sides and back of the head are commonly shaved with a straight razor.

IVY LEAGUE: Also known as a "Princeton." A very clean-cut style named for its popularity among men attending the "Ivy League" universities (Princeton, Harvard, Yale, et. al). Generally, the hair is cut very short all over, gradually getting slightly longer in front. Enough hair is left to part and comb neatly. Jerry Lewis wore an Ivy League haircut in "Nutty Professor."

LAYER CUT: A popular haircut which is performed entirely with shears. Hair is cut in uniform "layers" all over the head. The cut can be as long or short as desired and can be a very versatile cut.

MULLET: The origin of the term "mullet" has been traced back to the film "Cool Hand Luke." Apparently one of the guys calls people with long, shaggy hair "Mulletheads." The style is popular among soccer players and country music singers. Generally the hair is cut short on top and on the sides, with considerable length left in the back.

POMPADOUR: A longer version of the classic tapered haircut in which the hair is brushed back and secured with a liberal application of pomade. The pompadour was the signature haircut of Elvis and was quite popular by young "rebels" in the 1950s.

PRINCETON: Also known as a "Ivy League." A very clean-cut style named for its popularity among men attending the "Ivy League" universities (Princeton, Harvard, Yale, et. al). Generally, the hair is cut very short all over, gradually getting slightly longer in front. Enough hair is left to part and comb neatly.

SHAG: long layer cut that is cut using a razor to give the haircut a deconstructed (shaggy) look. This is an easy to maintain style and requires only a little product and a good shake to look great.

SKIN FADE: A faded or tapered haircut in which the sides and back have maximum scalp exposure. It is cut bald halfway up the head, then blended in to the top.

TAPERED NAPE: Hair at the back of the neck is graduated to zero length, leaving an exposed natural hairline. The advantage to a taper is that, as the hair grows out, the neckline remains natural and blended. This will give the haircut a fresher look longer than a blocked nape.

Haircuts By Numbers

A man's layer cut and a lady's layer cut are exactly the same, only with feminine or masculine lines. Men or women who wear a basic layer cut should be able to go to a barber or a cosmetologist.

As we discussed in a previous chapter, traditional men's haircuts are not usually a typical cosmetologist's preferred field of expertise. As I stated before, there are always exceptions to a rule and there are some who know how to taper the hair gradually. However, when a *typical* cosmetologist does a man's short haircut, they will usually use one of the plastic guards on the clippers to cut the sides and back. Sometimes they will also use a large clipper guard to cut the top. To a barber, it would be just as easy to cut the top with scissors. Let's take for example, a man who wants his hair cut above his ears and short on the sides and back, but has thick, full hair on top that he likes to comb over to the side. A *typical* barber would use a clipper and comb to cut the hair gradually and taper it up to the length at the crown. Then he would cut the top like a layer cut and blend it all in together. A *typical* cosmetologist would use a guard on their clipper and run it up about halfway, then use a bigger guard above that and then possibly use a really big guard to cut the top. I am putting emphasis on the word "typical" for a reason.

It's not to say that one method of cutting is better than the other. Many customers are perfectly satisfied with the haircuts done with the plastic guards. There are a lot of young men who have never had their hair cut any other way. They've never been taught or told the difference and often have never had their hair cut by a barber. So asking for a particular number for a haircut length seems perfectly normal.

To a traditional barber, that haircut is usually called a "fade" which is different than a "regular" haircut. To a barber, most men's haircuts are cut gradual from shortest on the hairline and gradually getting longer. It takes a lot of practice and many years of experience to do a really nice taper. A "fade" to a barber, is where the hair is cut by a blade (the same length—not gradually getting longer) up to where the head starts to round in, above the temple area, and then blended in from that point up to the top. The customer doesn't know the difference and therefore doesn't know how he wants it cut. He doesn't know any better.

If he combs his hair to the side, he most likely needs to leave it long enough so that the cowlick won't stick up and the hair will lie down flat. It is generally more pleasing to the eye if it is cut gradually getting longer, especially on the side the "part" is on. And it is usually easier for an experienced barber to cut it that way. The barber has a lot more control of the length he's cutting the hair to. With the blades and attachments, once the barber decides what blade to use, and cuts with it, it is cut. There is no putting it back.

Another potential problem is that the cosmetologist might tell the customer, "That's a #2 on the sides and a #6 on top. (Or whatever numbers being used) The customer loves to be able to give simple number directions like that. To them, it seems less complicated. However, now the problem is that same man walks into a barber shop and tells the barber, "I would like a #2 on the sides and a #6 on top." To a barber looking at the man in the chair, he has a "regular" haircut, and would most likely be more happy with the clipper over comb or scissor over comb, gradual tapered haircut. But the customer doesn't know the difference between a barber's tools and a cosmetologist's tools.

Now the barber is frustrated because he knows he can give this guy a better haircut doing it his own way, but this guy has just taken the free choice of tools to use out of his hands. He's asking the barber to use "training wheels" instead of applying his twenty or thirty years of experience and training. In other words, it's like the barber is capable of cooking this guy a gourmet meal and he wants him to make him a hot dog.

Then there is another problem. More than likely, the barber doesn't *have* a #6 plastic guard. The biggest blade on the Oster® is a #3 ½. Besides that, the plastic guards' numbers/sizes do not correspond to the same number/size on an Oster® clipper. If the barber were to listen and follow these instructions and use his Oster® #2 on the sides, it would be way shorter than the cosmetologist's #2 plastic guard. So now after the barber has explained all this to the man who really thought he was making things less complicated, the barber (*who's area of expertise is men's haircuts*) looks like an idiot who doesn't know how to do the haircut. Talk about frustrating!

Now let's take for example, a man who wants a buzz cut. That's where all the hair is about a 1/4" long all over the head. He goes into a sign—in type shop at the mall, and the stylist uses a plastic #2 on him and tells him to ask for that number when he comes for his next haircut. Then next month he goes into a barber shop and wants the same haircut. A "traditional" barber would use a #2 Oster® blade. The hair is cut way shorter than the plastic guard #2 and now the customer is mad at the barber.

It's really a shame that the makers of the plastic guards and the makers of the Oster® blades don't get together and make a "universal" number system, but they haven't. Until that day comes, this is a new and very frustrating challenge for the barbers. The barber would have to be psychic to know if the customer is giving them Oster® numbers or plastic guard numbers. I am not placing blame on the customer or on the cosmetologist, or on the barber. I am not looking to blame anyone. I just feel it is important for the customer to be aware of these differences in order to increase their odds of getting the haircut they want.

The customer would be much better off to stop trying to tell each person cutting their hair *how* to cut it. They should just tell the operator how they want their hair to look when it's finished, not the process of how to get it there, because what works for one operator doesn't always work for another. We all work differently. Even barbers and stylists within the same shop work differently and use different tools.

You should not assume to know if the operator is a barber or a cosmetologist according to their gender. Just like you can't assume the female who is wearing a lab coat in the hospital to be a nurse and the male wearing a lab coat in the hospital to be the doctor. Often these days, the female is the doctor and the male is the nurse. The same kind of thing has happened in the "hair" industry. There are plenty of female barbers and plenty of male cosmetologists. They can each work in either type of shop or salon. It doesn't mean they can't all do the same haircut. But they each do it a different way. It's best to leave the creative rights to the person doing the creating. Let each operator work with what they are comfortable working with. I think it is so odd in the first place that a customer would tell a professional what tools to use. I can't imagine telling my mechanic what tools to use, or my dentist or my surgeon. It's one of my biggest pet peeves.

The Process Of A Haircut

When a customer goes into a barber shop for a haircut, one of the barbers should greet them or acknowledge them in some way. If all the barbers are busy, the customer should take a seat in the waiting area, taking note of who is ahead of them in line. When it is your turn, you should wait until the barber calls for whoever is next. You should give the barber time to finish the customer they're working on, which includes collecting payment and saying good-bye, give them time to brush the hair off of their chair and their tools, and hold the chair for you. You wouldn't believe how many customers get up and come over to get in the chair as we're pulling the cape off the guy we're working on! Think about it. Of course we're not ready yet. The person in the chair usually wants to stand up and get a closer view, then they need time to gather their keys, glasses, hat, cane, purse, jacket etc. Then we walk together to the register and collect payment. Sometimes we have to wait while they write a check out. More often, it's cash, and we have to make change and then say thank you and goodbye.

Barbering is a messy business and there are laws we have to follow regarding sanitation. Once we walk back to our station, we have to blow or wipe the hair off the chair, dust the hair off our clippers, and get a clean comb for the next customer. Then we will turn the chair in the direction we like and ask for who is next. The barber should hold on to the chair firmly while a person is going to sit in it. Some barbers lock the chair and don't hold it, but when someone trips and is starting to go down, the lock doesn't do anything. The whole chair turns. Some people really struggle getting around the foot rest and just sitting down. All they have to do is turn around, place their hand on the arm of the chair, back up, and sit. But they try to get one foot inside the foot rest area and then get turned around, and that is a recipe for disaster. Others try to turn the chair toward the mirror. Even if the chair is locked, they will wrench it around with their hand before they sit down, which leads to chair repair.

Please do not turn the chair toward the mirror, or start giving us directions yet. We can turn you toward the mirror after we get the neck towel and the cape on you. It is much easier to reach our tools from within reach to the counter. As with any personal contact business, we follow sanitation rules, laws, and guidelines. The towel around your neck is so that the cape does not come into contact with your skin. We use the same cape for many customers. We will get you settled in the chair, take your things that you'd like for us to set on the counter for you, and then we will ask how you want your hair cut. If the barber doesn't turn you to face the mirror, and you have an overwhelming urge to look at yourself, you may ask to be turned around. For now, just simply sit down in the chair. Customers some-times will start giving us instructions before we are ready to listen. We like to give you our full attention and have a comb in our hand while you tell us what you want.

Think of going to the barber shop like when you go to a doctor: First the nurse or assistant comes in and gets you prepared for the doctor. We don't have a nurse or assistant, but we still have to put the towel and the cape on you, and get our tools clean and ready for a new haircut. It just takes a couple of minutes and then we'll be ready to talk to you. The barber will *always* ask you how you want it to be cut before he starts. Unless he's been cutting your hair every month for sev-eral years, I can not imagine *any* barber not asking the customer what they want before they start. Relax. We won't shave your head as soon as you're not looking or anything like that.

You should make sure your "part" is in the correct place before we start and that your hair is combed or brushed in the general direction that you normally wear it. A "part" is where you "split" or "separate" the hair in two directions. People part their hair on the left, on the right, in the middle, and in any other variation possible. Some comb or brush their hair straight back on top with no part. Others comb their hair straight down with no part. The hair in the front that lies on the forehead is called "bangs."

There are only so many directions you can comb your hair. You can comb it to the right. You can comb it to the left. You can comb it down on both sides. You can comb it back. You can comb it forward. You can make it stick up. We're not going to take it upon ourselves to change where you're hair is parted or how you wear it so you should come in for a haircut with your hair the way you normally wear it.

When it's time to give the barber your instructions, tell the barber the basic type of haircut you want, where you part it, how you comb it, and the general length you want it to end up. Tell us if you want a lot off or just a little off. Taking a little bit off all around while keeping the same basic style or haircut that you have is called a "trim." You can say "Just trim it up" if you're keeping the same haircut you had a month ago, and just want it maintained. Give directions for each part: (front, top, back, and sides) of your hair. If you're going for a major change, or we've never cut your hair before, a picture is ok to use.

If you need lengthy consultation, you should perhaps consider going to an appointment type salon. If you're doing the same cut you always get, we can pretty much see how it was cut. Basically, it's just maintenance.

If we've cut your hair before and did a good job, trust that we can do it again, but please refresh our memory and give us the same instructions you gave us before. If a barber does twenty three customers in a day, and works five days a week, he has more than likely cut somewhere around seven hundred haircuts since he last saw you. It's quite possible that he doesn't remember you. If we've been cutting your hair every month for the past ten years, it is safe to assume we remember what to do.

If you're going to a barber you've never used before, don't explain how the last person did it. Just tell us how you want it. Keep your directions as simple as possible. Most of the time, terms such as "short" "medium" and "long" work just fine. It's not rocket science. There is no need to spend ten minutes telling us what you want. Saying, "Just trim it up" works in a huge percentage of the time. Most haircuts are just maintenance.

As I've mentioned previously, I suggest that you refrain from saying directions in numbers or clipper guard/blade sizes unless you always go to the same barber. We all use different tools even among barbers in the same shop. You really don't need to tell an experienced barber the number or how the last person cut it. Just tell us what you want.

Everyone thinks their hair is more difficult to cut than the next guy's. That is generally not the case. Make sure the barber has understood your instructions clearly. They should repeat them back to you so that you know you are understood correctly. Once you know you're understood, you don't have to repeat them, especially after we've already started. It's kind of insulting to us that you think we're so dumb that we didn't hear you the first two times.

One thing I should mention here. The English language has a lot of words that have more than one meaning. One that causes barbers problems is when a customer says "I would like it cut over the ears." The word "over" can mean two different things. It can mean covering "over" the top of the ear, and it can mean cut "over" the ear, as in "above" the ear. It's best if you say "I would like it cut *above* my ear." or "I would like it cut to *cover* the top of my ear."

Once you are satisfied that the barber understands what you want, leave them alone and let them do their thing. A good barber with a little common sense can get started on a minimal amount of direction and ask questions along the way. For instance, we can start on the sides and ask, "medium on the sides?" As we cut the sides and work our way toward the back, we can ask "taper the back, or square it off?" Then when we get to the top, we can ask, "how much off the top?" etc.

The barber may or may not do it like your last barber or hairstylist did it. We all work differently, but most of us have a routine or an order of things we do in the same order for every customer. We develop habits. Hair-cutting is an art similar to painting a picture. One may start on the sides. One may start in the back. One may start on the top. One may start with the clippers. One may start with the scissors. One may start with the razor. One may start with the thinning shears. What works for one barber may not work for another. Whatever *that* particular barber is used to doing, is what they are going to be better at using. *Please do not* tell the barber what tools to use or how to go about his/her work. If that is the way he or she is used to working, that's what works best for that barber, to achieve the desired result. If you are confident that the barber understood what you want, just leave him alone and let him create it. You seriously handicap an artist if you tell him how to go about it. If you don't like it when they're done, ask them to make adjustments.

If we part your hair in sections as we go, please don't assume that we are thinking that you comb your hair that way. We're not ready to comb it the way you wear it while we're cutting it. We're just parting it to section it, so that we can pick the hair up with the comb.

Please don't tell us to cut the top shorter before we've even touched the top in first place. We can't do all parts of the haircut simultaneously. Give us more than three minutes to get to all parts of the haircut. Some barbers start on the top and work down. Some start at the neck and work up. There are a million ways to skin a cat. But my point is to please give us time. Wait until we get it to a certain point and then we'll ask if that's what you want. A smart barber will not cut your hair too short to start off with. We will cut a "rough draft" and then from there, we will "fine-tune" it. When we get to a certain point, we will show you and ask you if we need to make any adjustments. Maybe you want a little more off the top? Maybe one side looks a little thicker than the other? Maybe you have a tough wave you'd like us to work on a little more? We are not going to throw you out of the chair and make you keep this haircut. This is just a rough draft at this time. We can make as many adjustments as necessary at this point. We cannot make adjustments if we leave ourselves nothing to work with. If we've already cut the hair too short, there is not much we can do. We can only shorten the hair. We cannot make it longer or put it back.

Please don't tell us to take more off when we're just getting started. You might just ruin the haircut. We can come back to it, but let us use our own judgement as long as you feel we've understood you correctly. Rome wasn't built in a day, and we can't do a complete haircut in three minutes. Give us a few minutes. Some barbers like to "whittle" it down. It's like building a house: We build a foundation first. Then we build the walls. Then the roof. Then comes the electricity, decor, and landscaping. We can't build the roof if we haven't already built the foundation and the walls. Please just relax and let us get to a certain point before you start worrying about it. The bells and whistles will come last.

Once we get the desired length and movement, then we can adjust your sideburns where you want them, thin it out in the thick spots, work on the waves etc. If the barber has followed your directions, but you decide you want it shorter, that's not the barber's fault. If they've already spent fifteen to twenty minutes on your haircut, don't expect the barber to be cheerful about cutting the whole haircut shorter. We hate doing two complete haircuts for the price of one. We try our best to do what you say. If we misunderstood, didn't listen, or did it wrong, that's one thing. But if we've done what you said and then you changed your mind, that's another. It's one thing to make adjustments and cut a little more off here or there. It's another thing to start all over. People seem to think it's easier if we are taking a small amount off. It isn't any easier. We still have to go through all of the motions.

Last, but not least, we will ask if you want us to trim your eyebrows. We generally cut the hair in the ears as part of the haircut. I can't imagine anyone wanting us to leave the ear hairs, so we pretty much take it for granted that you want them cut. We usually ask first before we trim the eyebrows because there are some people who don't want them trimmed. The customer should probably ask for it if he wants his nose hairs cut. Most barbers will do it for you, but we don't want to embarrass you by asking.

We will not forget to shave your neck! You don't need to remind us. No man in the world likes the hair on his neck. It's part of the haircut. We realize it annoys you and we already know that you want us to shave it as low as possible. We will do the best we can. We're not in the business of shaving shoulders and backs so please don't expect us to. We will get the hair on the inside of your ears to the best of our ability. It is a hard place to get into. Please don't ask us to use scissors to get it. It's too easy to cut the customer. There is too high of a risk for injury.

About your sideburns.... If you shave every day, you are used to cutting your own sideburns. How often do you get them perfectly even? You actually have an advantage over the barber when it comes to getting your sideburns even. You can get your face right up close to the mirror and get the straight on view and then turn your face from left to right to see if they are even on both sides. When the barber cuts your sideburn, we stand to your side and look at one sideburn at a time. We can't stand right smack in front of you and hold your chin in our hand like a child's and turn your face from left to right to compare the two. We look at one side and then we walk around you and look at the other side. Or we put a finger tip on the bottom edge of each sideburn and look in the mirror, which is usually too far away to really see. Some men use their ears as a guide to where they cut their sideburns. Most peoples' ears are crooked. No joke. Some use the front view in the mirror to determine if they are even. Some men go by where their glasses lie. We have no idea which method you use, much less which is the best method to use. And, if your head is tilted in the slightest degree, the angle of our cut will be tilted upward or downward. We will do our best, but, what I don't understand is that men will go around with crooked sideburns every day of the month, but the day they get their hair cut, they want them to be perfect. I've seen men who could care less what their haircut looks like but then want me to spend ten minutes getting their sideburns perfect. You adjust them yourself the very next morning!

After we have finished making all the adjustments and have the hair cut to the length you want it, we will be ready to shave your neck. We can't get to the hair on your neck with the cape around your neck, so we generally wait until we are otherwise finished. The barber should, at this point, brush all the hair off your head and shoulders, open the cape, and shave your neck with the electric trimmers. Most barbers will try their best to not get the hair down your shirt. We are very much aware of how bad it itches. No one itches any more than we do! We wear it all day long. We give each customer the same attention to getting the hair off of them and do the best we can within reason.

After the neck is shaved, the barber should ask once again if everything is how you want it. Now is the time to say so if it's not short enough, or if it's still too thick, or if an area isn't laying right, or if something looks uneven. The barber won't comb your hair exactly like you do. I usually hand the customer my comb at this point and let them comb their own hair. Sometimes a person can tell more by the feel of it than by looking at it to know if they've gotten enough cut off. Run your fingers through it. Take a good look and make sure you're happy. There are people that come back a month later and say, "You left my hair too long last time!" It's not fair to blame the barber if wasn't cut short enough. We can always take more, and we will be happy to take more if you tell us to. There are also times when the customers make us take it shorter against our better judgement which may cause us to mess up a perfectly good haircut too. We know how long to leave cowlicks so that they don't stand up. We cut it just at the point of barely laying down and the person will want it cut shorter. Bangs tend to shrink up and look shorter after they dry, so be careful if you ask us to cut them shorter. It is ok to look at your haircut thoroughly. We will not be offended. You might notice that the bangs are crooked or something. It is entirely possible that we didn't cut them right. Have us take a good look and make sure they are straight. The barber may or may not offer you a mirror to look at the back. If you want to see it, ask for a mirror.

If the haircut meets your approval, at this point the barber will remove the cape and thank you for your patronage. It is customary to tip barbers and hair-stylists when they've done a good job. The barber may or may not remember if you're a "good tipper." We may or may not remember if you don't tip at all or tip sparingly. It is to your benefit if the barber likes you. Find a barber that you like and over the years you will develop a friendship of sorts with each other.

The Surly Barber

If the barber likes you, and is physically comfortable working on you, they will want you to come back and pay them to cut your hair every month. In a nutshell, the barber will "go the extra mile" and spend extra time giving you a perfect, precision haircut if you are not a huge pain in the neck, and you don't make our job harder than it needs to be. I apologize if I am not being politically correct, or if I am hurting anyone's feelings, but this chapter and some of the following chapters are going to be brutal at times. I am going to be honest and tell the customers exactly why they don't always get the service they would have liked.

These are the situations that tend to influence a barber to become "Surly," not only to that particular customer at that particular time, but also in an accumulative manner, in that some barbers tend to acquire a "surly" attitude in general. I'm sure that all professions have similar mood destroying situations that cause employees to become surly at times.

The bottom line is that if the barber likes you, and is comfortable working on you, they will look forward to seeing you come in every month. The barber will be happy to see you and will be delighted that you are his customer if you are friendly and respectful and at least *try* to cooperate. If you make the barber angry, insult them, do not cooperate, or are just a general pain in the neck, the barber has no *incentive* other than the price of the haircut to have to deal with it every month. If the price of the haircut is $13.00, the barber says to himself, "Is it worth $13.00 for me to ruin my day? Not only this day, but one day out of every month?" And he just might decide that it's not worth it.

I'm not meaning to scare anyone. Maybe some who read this book will be nervous that they are going to get a really bad haircut if they don't behave perfectly. Again, my intention is to increase the customer's odds of getting a good haircut. There are things that customers do, that they are not always aware of, that cause us physical discomfort and/or cause us to become defensive and surly.

It's not that we would give you a *"bad"* haircut anyway. To be honest, I don't even know how to do a *"bad"* haircut. Under normal circumstances, I wouldn't give someone a haircut that was shorter than what they asked for on purpose. Unless they make me re-cut the haircut several times, in which case I will most likely cut it very short. I take a lot of pride in my work, and I think most barbers and hairstylists do so also. I wouldn't leave the haircut unfinished, but I wouldn't want to build a following of customers who make me cut their hair three times either.

I certainly can't speak for all barbers. Some have more patience than others. I can only speak for myself. But common sense should tell you that if we have a customer in our chair who is a pain in the neck in some way or will not cooperate and is causing us physical discomfort we will get the job done as quickly as we can get away with, and perhaps not spend enough time fine-tuning the haircut and making it perfectly even. And we may perhaps get an attitude and become surly. If we like the person in the chair, and we are physically comfortable, it's more likely that we might have a conversation, ask about their family, get to know them, and generally piddle around with their hair until it looks it's best.

When I have a person in my chair and they sit crooked, or won't hold still, I try to correct them nicely. I will ask them to please sit nice and straight. If they correct themselves and try to cooperate, then we will get along fine and I will do my best. However, there are many times when I have asked a customer to sit straight and they look at me like I've insulted them. Or like I am asking way too much of them if they can't be properly comfortable. I understand that getting a haircut is very relaxing, but it is important to sit in such a way as to make it comfortable for the barber also. The customer only has to be in the chair for ten to fifteen minutes. The barber has to work with it for many hours a day. Barbers have many common occupational aches and ailments that are most often from compensating with their own posture so as not to have to require their customers to sit correctly. I'm sorry, but if my back is killing me and I've tried to get the customer to sit right and they won't, I will indeed get a bit annoyed and possibly even surly. I will try to get the job done quickly and I will not be as friendly. Again … I can only speak for myself.

The thing I think about is: "Do I really want to cut this guy's hair every month?" While we all need money, a $12.00 haircut once a month that causes me pain or aggravation that could even possibly lead to medical absence from work, is not worth it. Many barbers have chronic neck, shoulder, wrist and back problems from not making their customers sit properly. I feel that people have to sit straight in the optometrist's chair, in the dentist's chair, and in just about every other personal service experience. Why should they not expect to have to sit straight for the barber? Sitting straight increases the odds of getting a good haircut for several reasons. One is because the barber is more likely to take extra time on you and will look forward to cutting your hair again if he is comfortable. Another is the simple geometry of hair-cutting. If your head is on crooked, it will mess up the angles of the haircut.

Alignment

Please try not to cross your legs during the haircut! Most barbers feel intimidated to ask their customer not to cross their legs, so they just deal with it in discomfort and do the best they can. I feel that we are not doing the future of the business of barbering any good when we do that. I think we should tell our customers that it's important to sit straight and encourage them to do so. Ironically, barbers and most parents will tell small children to sit straight, but grown men don't seem to think it's important, and barbers feel funny asking grown men to sit straight.

When you cross your legs, your body leans to one side and one shoulder is lower than the other. It makes cutting a level line very difficult to do. It messes up our sense of direction. And it causes the barber *much* physical discomfort. When you cross your legs, your body is closer to the edge of the chair on one side, and further away on the other side. It makes your head sit at an incorrect angle from your shoulders. On the one side, the barber has to lean back to hold the hair at the correct angle and to see what he or she is doing. The barber's hips are then tucked in and their legs are bent in an uncomfortable manner.

(Illustration # 22 leaning toward barber)

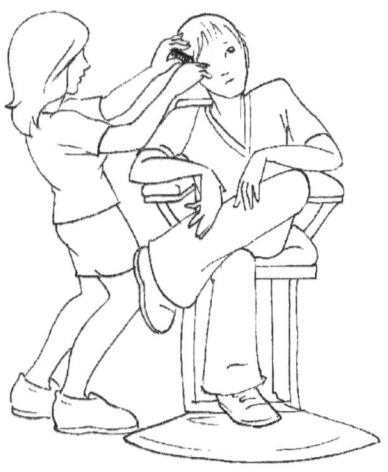

On the other side of the customer, the barber can barely reach your head! (**Ill. # 23**) Unless, of course, you have a very tall barber with very long arms. If you have a female barber or a short barber, chances are good that they don't have a long reach. If you have a female barber, she also has breasts and if she leans her body too close to the chair in order to reach your head (on the far away side) she will have to touch her bosom to your shoulder! I cannot stress enough how much it hurts the barber's back/body at the end of a busy day, if people don't cooperate and sit straight in the chair. I know it's asking a lot, but please be considerate of the barber's comfort and don't sit in the chair as if you're going to crack open a beer and turn the television set on! The barber will give you a much better haircut if he or she is not in pain or discomfort and as I've mentioned previously, it also changes the geometrical angles that we're holding the hair. In the following illustration, notice that if the barber pulls the hair from the center of his head toward herself, it will not be cut at 90 degrees off his head. It will over-direct the hair.

It seems to be a natural instinct that everyone wants to tilt their head away from us. If we were to tilt your head in any way, we would more likely tilt it *towards* us, to make it easier to reach and to see what we're doing. When the head is tilted or turned away from us, it makes it hard for us to reach and to see what we're doing. It's very important for us to be able to *see* what we're doing. We also need to be able to adjust the angle of your head according to what area we're working on. If we're working on the neckline, we will move your head downward, (chin on chest) so that we don't have to lean back and so that we can see what we're doing. If we're working on the side, we need to be able to reach your head with ease. Please don't tilt it away from us or turn it left or right. If you are facing the mirror, please don't turn your head left or right to see what we're doing. It is always best to just sit with your head straight unless the barber pushes your head or asks you to move it a certain way.

Please don't try to help us in any way. We have learned how to do this process all by ourselves, and it makes our job much harder when you try to help. If we want you to tilt your head in any way, we will simply push it gently in the direction we want or ask you to do it.

Illustration # 23 leaning away from barber

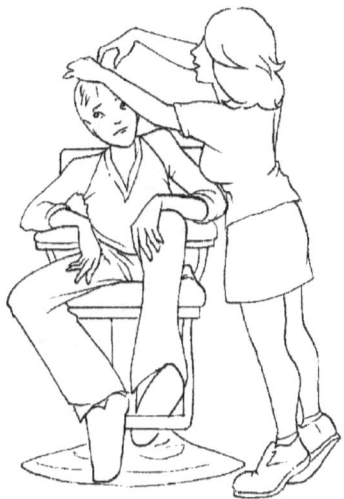

Please try to keep your chin up. Please do not be lazy and sit with your chin on your chest, watching the hair fall or sleeping. We are usually standing behind the chair to cut the top. If you tilt forward, it's harder for us to reach and to see what we're doing.

There are people who think they are doing us a favor by angling their heads in a certain way, or tilting their head down, or sitting a certain way.

Or they will try to anticipate where we're going and tilt their heads this way or that way, as we're moving around them. This *totally* drives us mad. While we appreciate their good intentions, and we know they are actually trying to help us, this actually is exactly backwards of helping us. Really, we just want your head to be straight and level, unless we tilt it a certain way ourselves. The neck is an awesome part of the human body. It has amazing flexibility and freedom of movement. There are several different ways we can turn and tilt our heads.

Illustration # 24 chin on chest

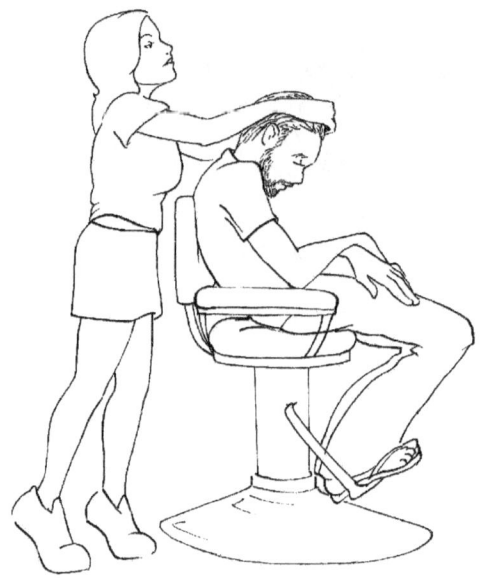

We can turn it left to right.

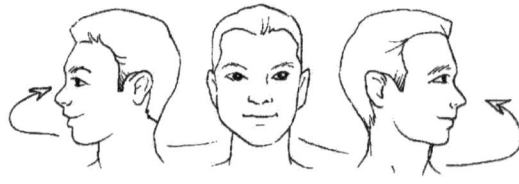

We can tilt it shoulder to shoulder.

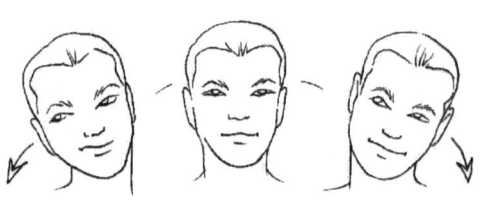

We can tilt it up and down.

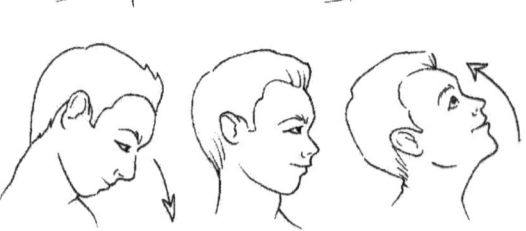

Illustration # 25 head range of motion

It's very important to keep your head still and straight forward. I cannot emphasize this enough. Customers often cause us to mess up their haircut by not keeping their head straight. People don't seem to realize that if their shoulders are crooked, it messes up our sense of what is level and what is not level.

STRAIGHT   CROOKED   RESULT

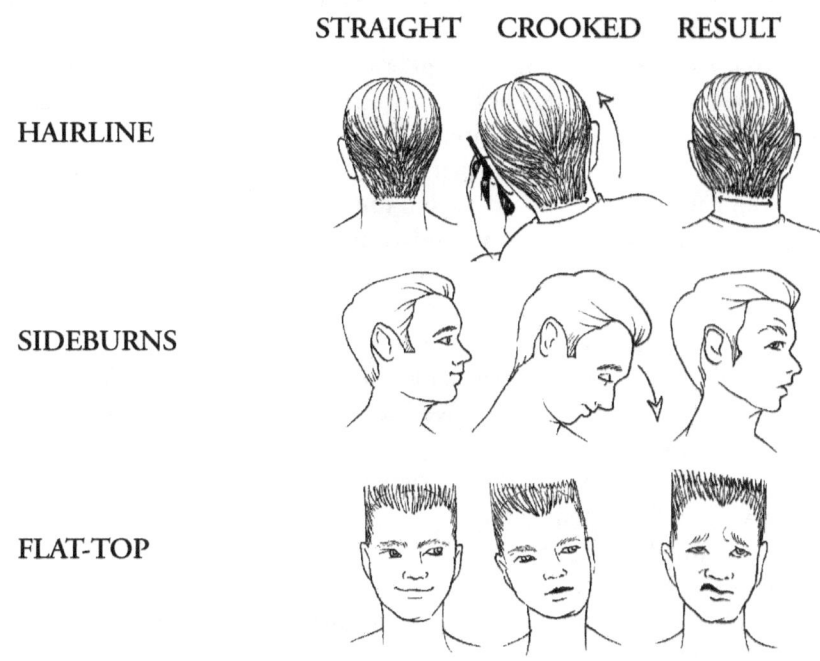

HAIRLINE

SIDEBURNS

FLAT-TOP

Illustration # 26 crooked heads crooked cuts

As you can see from the above illustrations, if we cut a straight line on the neckline, unaware that the head is not on straight, when the subject sets his head straight his neckline will not be level. Think of it like painting or drawing a picture. We have to draw a straight line across the neck.

If we cut the sideburn in a straight line, using our natural world (the ceiling and the floor) as our guidelines, and the subject has his head tilted downward, (chin on chest) when he lifts his head straight again, the sideburn will be cut on an angle whereby the line is pointed downward toward the ear. Likewise, if he tilts his head back, to look up, the line will be tilted into a pointy sideburn like "Spock."

If we are cutting a "flat-top" haircut, and we are unaware that our subject has his head tilted, we could finish the whole haircut before realizing we made him look like "Gumby!" Once the corners are cut off on a flat-top, there is no fixing it. If the corners get cut off, the haircut can only be turned in to a "buzz" cut or "crew cut."

Some people have a tendency to want to look at the barber's eyes while talking. It's natural to have eye contact when speaking to someone, but we can't cut your hair that way. We only have so much time to work on you, and we cannot work on your haircut if we have to stop and look you in the eye.

Keep your arms inside the chair and under the cloth. Some people want to sit with their elbow outside the edge of the armrest. We have to stand there and we don't want to brush up against your elbow.

Another thing you should know is that while we do like to see you smile, when you smile, your ears go up. If we are cutting the hair around your ears while you are smiling, you will have a space around your ears once they relax back into place. The same thing applies to raising your eyebrows while we are cutting your bangs. When you have a surprised or questioning expression on your face, or if you are trying to look at your bangs being cut, your eyebrows go up. We use the eyebrows as a guide to where to cut the bangs. If we cut the bangs while your eyebrows are up, they will be shorter than we had intended once the eyebrows relax back into their natural place.

When you wiggle around in the chair, there is great a potential that one of two things could very well happen: (1) You get your skin cut. (2) You get a shorter haircut than we intended to give you. No matter which tool the barber is using to cut your hair—whether it's scissors, clippers, or razor etc., they are all quite capable of cutting the skin. It is much more difficult than the average person thinks it is, to *not* cut a customer's skin during the course of a haircut. Cutting the hair around the ears is one of the most difficult areas as is any time when we are cutting the hair flat against the skin. Most people don't realize that when they move their hands and feet, their head wiggles.

A lot of people seem to instinctively move their heads around when they talk. It's extremely difficult for us to work on a moving target. We pick the hair up with our comb (or fingers) and we aim for a spot with the cutting instrument. If the spot we are aiming for moves closer or further away than we're aiming for, we'll either cut it deeper than we intended to, or miss it all together and cut our finger. It makes us have to cut the surrounding hair shorter in order to blend in the boo boo, which results in a shorter haircut than we intended. In a worst case scenario, we may cut the person's skin.

The Circle Of Life

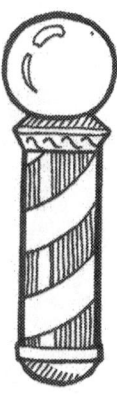

Over The Years

When you find a barber or a barber shop that you like and you go there regularly for haircuts, you will get to know your barber and the other barbers in the shop and they will get to know you as well. As you sit in the chair, the barber and the customer talk and get to know each other. It's amazing how much information is passed around in a barber shop. The top news stories are discussed, sports are discussed, the stock market, the neighborhood golf game, current events, the weather, children's local sports and so forth. If anything is going on in town, it will be a topic of the barber shop. Barber shops were once gathering places for men to talk to each other and catch up on the latest news. Beauty salons were once the same for women. A lot of customers in small towns know each other. They play golf together and their kids know each other from school.

Over the years, you get to know each other. Think of the old barber who's worked in his same little town since he was a young man. He's watched children grow up, and has seen his classmates grow old. In many cases, the barber's dad was a barber too! If a barber stays at the same job for several years, they get to watch the cycle of life in a profound way. Let's say a customer gets married and has a baby. The customer has kept the barbers informed of the progress of the pregnancy all along and has a healthy baby with a full head of hair. Eventually he brings the baby in to get his first haircut. A month or so later, they come back and this time the boy doesn't cry and he isn't so frightened of the barber. The barber has remembered his name. The boy tells the barber how old he is and the barber asks the boy what he likes to do for fun. A new relationship is formed. Each month, the boy is getting older and more mature. A few months go by and the mom is pregnant again! Another haircut in a few months! The next thing you know, the boy is going into high school, and the parents are bringing in their aging parents for haircuts, because they don't drive much anymore. Eventually, that baby boy is now a young man starting his own family, bringing his boys in for haircuts. And the cycle goes on and on.

Baby's First Haircut

Babies' first haircuts are extremely hard to do. You should look for an experienced barber for your child's first haircut. Inexperienced barbers are frightened that they might cut the child if they wiggle and it makes them very nervous. Elderly barbers have a hard time bending and reacting quickly and it's especially hard on their backs and their nerves. The kid is wiggling around and crying. When a child cries, they get a runny nose and their face gets moist with tears, and then the hair clippings get stuck all over their face. Then they become even more irritated and miserable! There are many things the parents can do and say that can make our job even harder. There are also many things a parent can do or say to make our job much easier and much less traumatic for the child.

Children are naturally scared of the barber. To be honest, they have good reason to be! We work with very sharp tools and it is extremely hard to *not* cut the child's skin if he is moving around. Even the slightest movement by any age customer can cause the barber to miss their aim and cut the skin. It's a very scary job for the barber and for the child too. The parent, and the barber can make the difference between the haircut being a traumatic event or a fun event.

I have some suggestions of do's and don't's before the time actually comes when you take a child in to the barber for his first professional haircut. No offense to the beauticians/hairstylists, but I feel it is better to take small boys to a barber shop in most cases. Barbers specialize in men's and boys' haircuts. The boy is in a masculine setting and feels like a "big boy." The barber shop has things in the decor that are more likely to appeal to the boy's masculine psyche.

But either way, Mom or Dad have decided to get the boy his first professional haircut. If the boy is old enough to understand words, explain to him that it's time for him to have his hair trimmed up to make it look good. Try to refrain from saying he's going to get his hair *cut*. Small children just learning to speak English have begun to make word associations. They may hear the word *cut* as something that is going to hurt and possibly cause bleeding. Explain, before you go to the barber shop, that it will not hurt. Small children don't understand how the hair has no feeling in it when it's cut. Their hair is a part of their body and they think it will hurt just like when they cut their finger. Have the boy go with his dad when his dad goes for a haircut so that he can watch and see that nothing is hurting his dad. Let the barber know that you are preparing the boy for his first haircut.

Some children are frightened by the cape. Explain to the boy that the barber puts a cape on Daddy to keep the hair clippings from falling on him and that's it is ok. When the barber starts cutting the hair, let the boy know that it doesn't hurt. "See? Daddy isn't crying!" usually gets a good laugh out of the other people in the shop. It's nice if the barber gives the boy a lollipop or something nice so that the boy associates the barber shop with "nice" people.

So now the day has come for the boy to get his first haircut. Tell him what a big boy he is now and how good it will feel to have his hair trimmed up. Make it a special day! Some barber shops offer a "first haircut" certificate and will cut a piece of hair for you to put in their baby book if you ask them. It's ok to take a picture if you want to. I personally, believe in the bribe and reward method. Tell the boy he will get a lollipop or ice cream or something special if he is real good. Tell him not to cry and to hold very still. I strongly suggest bringing a cookie or dry cereal, or some other favorite non-sticky treat to give to the child *during* the haircut. It keeps their mind off what is happening and usually distracts them if they start crying. Once you have decided that this is the day to get the boy's hair cut, it's best (in my opinion) if you stick to your guns. If they cry and the parent gives in and doesn't make them do it, they are usually even worse the next time. In most cases, it is not possible to do a perfect haircut on a baby the first time. It's more important just to get them used to the process and not to be afraid of it. You're doing good if you get through the first haircut with a minimum of trauma.

Different barbers do things differently, but I have found some things over the years of my experience that seem to work well with first haircuts. The cape seems to scare small children. Rather than get them all upset over it, if they are scared, I feel it is best to take their shirt off and cut the hair without using the cape. If you do the haircut without the cape, but leave the child's shirt on, the hair gets stuck in the fabric and pokes at them and causes great discomfort which they perceive as torture. The towel we have to put around their neck is itchy and uncomfortable. We are supposed to use them by law, because of sanitation issues. We can't let the cape touch the customer's skin. I find that often the children are more comfortable just letting the hair clippings fall onto their bare skin. They also tend to dislike not being able to see and to use their hands when they are under the cape, so if I do use the cape, I show them where their hands are and let them take them out.

What works for one situation isn't going to work for all. If the child doesn't mind the cape, then by all means, use it! If he doesn't want his shirt off, leave it on. It's not worth getting them all upset over. In any case, the barber should put a cape around the parent's shoulders, because the hair will be falling all over them.

Before the barber starts to cut anything, what I believe helps a lot, is for the barber to explain to the child that the clipper will only cut the hair and will not cut the skin. It's a fairly complex idea for a young child to understand, if you think about it. If it cuts the hair, why wouldn't it cut the skin? I like to explain it to the child and then let them or their parent touch the blade of the clipper to show them that it won't hurt. Let him feel how they feel against his skin. They usually get a big kick out of how they "tickle!" You can make it fun. Even though the clippers are noisy and tend to scare the child at first, I feel they are the best tool to start out with, because (1) They (generally) can't cut the skin. (2) They are faster. The faster the barber can get the job done, the better. Their patience doesn't last long and the more hair that falls on them, the more uncomfortable and upset they become. It's very important that the barber works quickly.

If the child gets upset over the clippers and still doesn't want to get his hair cut, this is the time to try the "cookie trick." I like cookies because they seem to comfort the child, it makes them happy, it gets their mind off the haircut torture going on, and they're not sticky. Lollipops and other sticky candies are not good to use during the haircut. The mess is unbelievable! I have used them in a pinch, but, the child won't keep it in his mouth with his lips wrapped completely around it and the hair will fall all over it and stick to it. The child will drool when it's in his mouth and the hair will stick to the drool. He will have his hand exposed to the hair falling, in order to hold the stick. Then the hair will stick to his sweaty little hands. Then he will use his hands or the cape (with all the hair on it) to wipe his face and get the hair in his eyes, up his nose, and in his mouth. Meantime the drool will be dripping all over the barber's cape, rendering it useless for the rest of the day. After this whole ordeal, the barber will have to spend ten minutes cleaning up the mess. Cookies, cereal or "smarties" are perfect. Barber shops usually have a candy jar, but they might only have lollipops, so it's a good idea for the parent to bring something.

When the child gets uncomfortable, they start crying and the parent feels like the child is going to hate them. It's hard on the parent, particularly the moms. Some barbers try to get the child to sit by himself in a booster chair because it is very difficult for most barbers to cut the child's hair while the parent is holding them. Personally, I feel it's best for the parent to hold the child for the first few haircuts, until they get used to the idea and it no longer frightens them. However, I have a suggestion for a way to hold a child that works really well for the barber and makes the child feel more secure: Hold the child as if you are hugging them, with their body against your chest and the left side of their face against your left shoulder. (**Illustration # 27**)

Illustration # 27 Baby Right Side

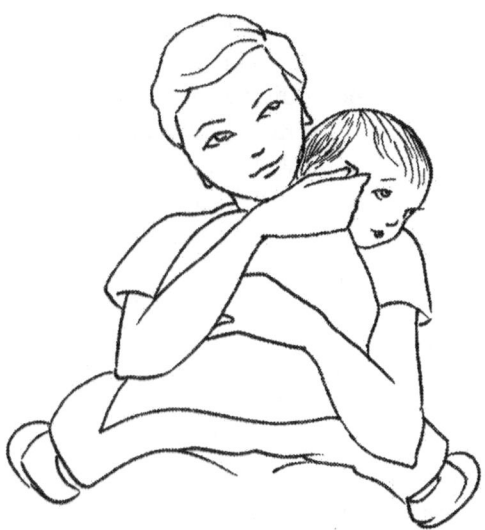

In this position, the child feels like he is being comforted. The barber has access to the whole side of his head. It's easier for most barbers to start on the right side of the subject's head and move around to the other side because we hold the comb in our left hand and the cutting instrument in our right hand. The parent can then take their left hand to hold the child's head firmly against their shoulder. He may cry because he doesn't like his movements restrained, but it's better to hold him with a firm hand, preventing movement so that the barber doesn't cut the child, than to feel bad because the boy is crying. Please hold his head very firmly, preventing all movement. The parent can also take the fingers of their right hand and hold the child's ear down, so that it is out of the barber's way, preventing the possibility of cutting the ear. While the clippers themselves won't actually cut the skin, it's very easy to pinch the skin between the comb and the clipper blades. The barber only has two hands. We hold the comb in one hand and the clippers in the other hand. We don't have another hand to hold the ear out of the way, which is always one of our most difficult tasks.

You certainly don't have to help the barber. He or she can manage on their own, and have more than likely never had a parent offer to do this before. It's just a trick I've learned over the years that I feel helps a lot by accomplishing three things: (1) It makes it easier/safer/faster for the barber to do his work. (2) It makes the child feel more secure and protected. (3) It makes the parent feel more secure that the barber isn't going to cut the child's ear and gives the parent a way to participate and comfort their child. The parent can say to the barber, "Do you want me to hold his ear down?" while showing him/her what you mean. If the barber is not receptive to the idea, I don't recommend pushing it. The barber may not be comfortable with it. I discovered this little trick by accident one day when a mom just did it! At first I felt weird about it, but then I discovered what a wonderful thing it is to do it this way! I also do the same thing on elderly gentlemen who have sensitive ears due to skin cancer and thin skin. I ask them to go ahead and hold their ear down for me. Sometimes I have young boys do it too. It makes them feel safer, and gives them something to do. Kids usually love a chance to help.

While you are holding the baby this way, I find it easiest to do the first side (the right side of his head) and go as far toward the back of his head as possible, and then have the parent turn the boy to the other shoulder. Place the boy's head with the right side of his face against the parent's right shoulder and do the same thing on this side, using your left hand to hold the ear down while firmly holding his head against your shoulder. (**Illustration # 28**) Then I work from the front of his left side and go as far toward the back as possible. You'll have to make some positioning adjustments so that the barber can get to the back. For the front, I usually just have the parent set the child on their lap facing out and hold the child's head firmly with their hands on either side of the child's head. (**Illustration # 29**)

Illustration # 28 Baby Left Side

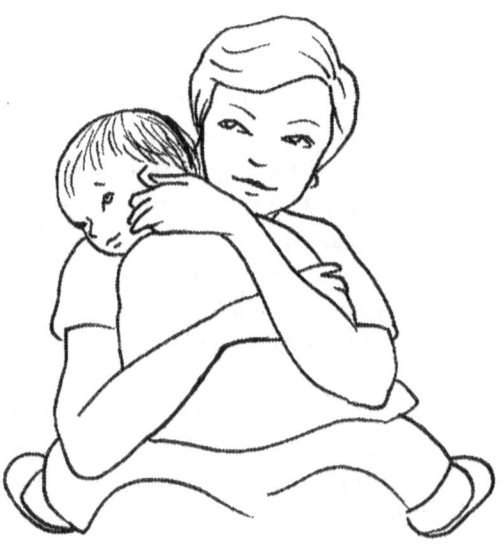

Illustration # 29 Baby facing barber

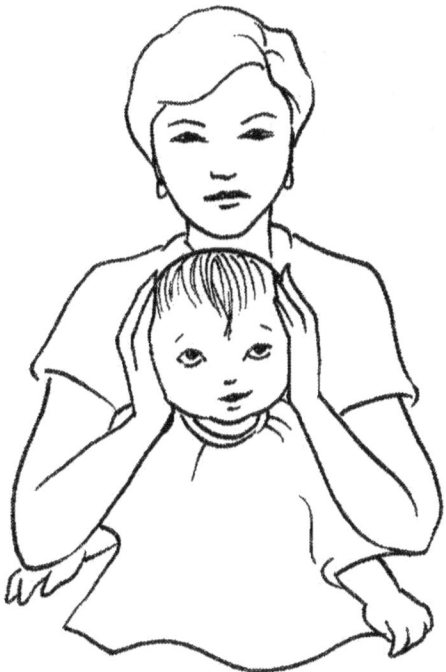

In the case of exceptionally frightened children, sometimes the parent or the barber simply gives up. Sometimes it's just impossible to do without bordering on child abuse. If you have one of these children, I suggest that you simply try again in a few weeks. In the meantime, try showing them that it doesn't hurt. I had one exceptionally tough case a few years ago. The mom was at her wit's end trying to get the boy to get his hair cut. He was absolutely terrified of it. Finally, one day, she carried him in sound asleep on her shoulder. I did the whole haircut on this little guy and he never woke up! He got a good haircut and it was quite easy for me. The mom just positioned his little sound asleep head to where I could get access and he never woke up. We did his next few haircuts the same way. Sometimes he would open his eyes and look around, but then he would go right back to sleep. He eventually grew out of his fright and was fine. Children generally sleep quite sound. I recommend this as a last resort. It may or may not work, but is worth a try.

When the haircut is as good as it's going to get, or the child has had enough, (whichever comes first) the barber should brush the hair off and put some powder on the boy's neck. Powder soothes their skin, absorbs the moisture, and makes the hair brush off easier. Most barber shops will give the boy a lollipop or something and try to be friends now. If the barber did a good job and went out of their way to try to be patient and understanding, they deserve a generous tip. First haircuts are as hard on the barber as it is for the child and the parent. They are very hard to do and they require a lot of skill and experience.

Little Guys

After a few haircuts with the parent holding the child, and they've become used to the process, we graduate them to the booster chair phase. Toddlers and small children still find it a challenge to sit still, but they will eventually. In this phase, the parent still has a lot of influence over whether the child gets a good haircut or not. It's nearly impossible at this age to do a complicated haircut. Keep it basic. Most little boys just get a "regular boy's haircut." The barber will ask the boy to sit still if he's moving too much, but we only have so much control over your child. If you see that the boy is not cooperating, it is appropriate for the parent to admonish the child and make him behave. In this phase, I suggest offering the lollipop reward only if the child has been good. A parent can offer some things for motivation such as not being allowed to do something the child really wants to do if he doesn't behave.

At this age, the child cannot be expected to sit perfectly still. It's important for the barber to move quickly. The longer the child has to sit still, and the more hair that gets on his skin, the more upset they become. Children at this age still like to see their hands, although it is best if they will keep their hands under the cape if they will. Otherwise, the hair falls on their hands and they will inevitably wipe their face with them getting the hair in their mouth and eyes and nose. When they have their hands under the cape, they will often use the cape to wipe their face which is even worse! *Every* child seems to do this! We explain to them that the cape is "dirty," it has the hair clippings all over it, and to take their hands out to wipe their face, but they will still do it again and again.

Some barbers do not want the parent to stand right at their chair while they're cutting the child's hair. They may want the parent to go sit down and leave them alone. If the parent wants to stand there and help, please don't stand right on top of us. Make sure you stand out of the barber's way. We're looking at the hair we're cutting, not at our feet. If you crowd us, we could trip. And please don't blow the hair off the child's face and into ours. Parents don't realize that our face is right behind the child's. They go to blow the hair off the kid's nose and it blows right into our eyes.

The barber should be able to handle it all on their own for the most part, but it's helpful if the parent will remind the child to sit still and sit straight and sometimes it helps if the parent provides distraction and a focal point. "Look straight at Mommy!"

The hardest part of the haircut at this age is clipping the hair on the neck and the neckline. Kids at this age usually have very ticklish necks. When we use the clipper on their neck, they get tickled and scrunch up. It's very hard for the barber to move quick enough to cut the hair and avoid injury. The clippers/trimmers generally won't cut the skin, but they can sure hurt if we jab them in the head with them, or if they slam their head into them. I recommend bringing a small toy along too. They seem to like to hold something in their hands while they get their hair cut. It will also give them something to play with while you are waiting for your turn. Some barber shops have toys or a television to watch, but many shops have nothing to entertain children. I like to keep small dinosaurs and action figures to use if the need arises, and I keep something interesting to look at on my counter.

Try to time the haircut when the child is not tired or grumpy. Nap-time is not a good idea. If the child doesn't want a haircut and you give up, just try again in a couple of days. In the meantime, you can try to bribe or cajole or discipline him into it. The barber only has so much time to try. Make sure the child understands where they are going and what's going on before you get there.

The Big Boys

Big boys are learning to comb their own hair and starting to have preferences of their own. Whether you or the child decides what kind of haircut to get, please make sure you have decided before getting to the barber shop. We can't solve your arguments for you. It's ok to let the child explain what he wants to the barber. We can usually figure out what he's trying to say, and if we don't understand, we will ask you to interpret.

Generally, there is a popular style that the little boys are getting, or it's a regular haircut combed differently. Kids at this age like to experiment with hair products such as gel and hair-spray. If there is a large amount of gel in the hair, the hair becomes so slippery and slimy that it's hard to hold on to and it feels extremely gross in our fingers. Then when we get the gel on our fingers, we can hardly hold on to our clippers without dropping them. A sink is not always nearby to rinse our hands. We can manage if there is only a small amount of it in the hair, but he will get a better haircut if the hair is clean. Please try to bring them with their hair clean and without sticky stuff in it, if possible. Preferably not wet though. The clippers are not designed to cut wet hair. It gums them up, and we can't see the blend as well. We can manage if there is only a small amount in it, but he will get a better haircut if the hair is clean and dry. Sticky stuff also causes us to pull and tug on the hair which causes discomfort for the child. Big kids tend to be the most cooperative customers. They generally sit straight and still. They are generally polite and well mannered.

Head lice tends to be a problem in the preschool and elementary school age kids. Head lice is not something a person gets because they are dirty. On the contrary, they prefer clean hair. Lice are transferred from person to person on hairbrushes, combs, hats, clothes and direct contact. Check the child's scalp periodically. The lice themselves are very hard to see, especially in dark colored hair. They are smaller than a flea and almost transparent. The lice lay eggs on the hair shaft called "nits." They look like little tiny beads on the hair near the scalp and they don't come off when you pull them. If you suspect your child may have lice, *please* don't bring them to the barber shop. They are highly contagious. By law, we are not allowed to cut their hair until they've been treated and are completely lice and nit free. We typically won't notice them in the hair until we have already started. We have to stop at that point and cannot finish the haircut. The child is humiliated when we have to call the parent over and explain that we can't finish the haircut because the child has lice. There are several treatments available in most drug stores and general stores. "RID®" is the most common brand. You have to treat the hair with the product twice and use a fine-toothed comb to remove all the dead nits. By law, we are not allowed to cut the hair if there are nits in it, even if they are dead nits.

Teenagers

Teenagers tend to start getting fussy about their hair. They like to do radical things with it to shock their parents. National and world wide haircutting trends are created by teenagers. Teenagers will typically want the opposite of whatever trend was popular in their parent's youth. If the parents like short hair, a teenager will likely wear it long and visa-versa.

Teenagers are perfectly capable of telling the barber how they want their hair cut, but they most likely won't want it like the parents want it. Often, parents come in with their teenage kids and wait until the kid is in the barber's chair to decide what kind of haircut to get. The boy tells the barber what he wants and then the parent says "No, I think it should be this other way." Then they start arguing and expect the barber to mediate between them. This puts the barber in a bad position which takes up valuable time. We don't want to make either of you unhappy, and we don't know who to listen to! We cannot stand around doing nothing while you argue over the haircut. While it would seem reasonable to assume that we would just do what the parents say, we really can't do that. The kid is our customer too. From what I've seen, when all is said and done, the parents usually lose the battle and give in anyway.

When the parent and the teenager are in disagreement, I will usually try talking them both into doing what I call "The Compromise Special" so that we can at least get started in some direction. We can make modifications as we go along or, preferably after we get it to the "rough draft" level. For instance, if the teenager wants his bangs hanging down in his eyes, and the parent wants them cut above his eyebrows, I would cut it so that it's right at the eyebrow, somewhere between what she wants and what he wants. If the parent wants his ears exposed and the kid wants his ear covered, I would suggest just covering the tip of the ear and go from there. We can always make adjustments after we get it somewhere close to the desired end result.

It is best if you decide on what kind of haircut to get before you get to the barber shop though. Not only is it time-consuming for the barber to have to be a mediator, but I would imagine this would be embarrassing to the parent and the child to argue about it in front of the entire barber shop. And please, don't push the responsibility onto the barber by asking us what we think looks best. It's not our job to tell you how to wear your hair. The barber may like completely different styles than you do. The barber's favorite haircut on a man could very well be a mohawk or something crazy like that.

Teenagers tend to like to use hair products too. Again, someone should teach them that they shouldn't use gel or other slimy products in their hair if they plan to go to the barber that day. If they go to a salon where they wash the hair first, it isn't a problem.

Teenagers also seem to go through a poor posture phase where they like to sit all scrunched down in the chair. They set their butt on the front edge of the chair, instead of all the way back against the back of the chair, where it should be in order to sit up straight. It's very uncomfortable for us to work on someone sitting this way. They need to sit with their rear end against the back of the chair, with their back straight, so that we can bend their head down when we need to. The other thing teenagers typically do, is sit straight but with their chin on their chests. It's like it's entirely too much work for them to hold their head up. Quite often in my experience, I've taken their head in my hands and brought it up where it's supposed to be, and as soon as I get back to the haircut they will drop it right back down again. This is extremely frustrating to the barber. So then I explain to them that it is important and ask them to please keep their head up, but they will keep on dropping it down again. The end result is that the barber gets aggravated with them because it is very frustrating to keep having to correct them and it hurts out bodies to work this way. If we worked like that all day long, we would be exhausted and sore when we got home. Therefore, it is probable that the barber might try to hurry up and get finished. And perhaps not want to cut this kid's hair again. What would you do if you were the barber?

Some teenagers are allowed to go to the barber shop by themselves. If you let your child come alone, expect us to cut it the way he tells us to cut it. Make sure that you trust the kid to not do anything crazy like a mohawk or something of that nature, if you're opposed to that kind of thing.

Parents should teach teenagers that it's customary to tip barbers and hairstylists and teach them what is an appropriate amount to tip. Teaching them to come in with their hair reasonably clean, to sit straight and still, and to be polite is also greatly appreciated.

Mid-Life Issues

From the time we are born, until the time when we die, our hair is changing with age. In the early stages of life, the hair is maturing to a more coarse texture and growing in density. As boys go through adolescence and puberty, they start to get facial hair. In mid-life years, men typically start to become grey. Most men also start losing their hair. Many men become completely bald. Hair starts to grow in the ears and the nose and the eyebrows start to grow long. They ask us: "Why do I have hair growing in my ears?" There is no tactful way for us to answer that question truthfully. The simple honest truth is that it's part of the process of male aging. Please don't make us tell you you're getting old! I don't know how men barbers feel about it, but every time I hear a man ask me that question, I want to tell them about all the wonderful signs of aging women get. We may not get hair in our ears, but we have plenty of our own issues including mustaches and sagging body parts. Aging takes it's toll on our beauty, whether male or female. There is only so much the barber can do.

Premature balding can be quite traumatic to a young man. Unfortunately, the barber cannot make the hair thicker. We are quite sympathetic. However, the majority of adult men are in some phase in the process of balding, not the minority, therefore the majority of the haircuts we do are for balding men.

Some men grow it long and try to hide the bare spot, sometimes referred to as a "comb-over" while some men would rather just cut it short or buzz it entirely off. They come up with all sorts of creative ways to comb their hair to hide their bald spots. I had a customer at one time who would part his hair about a half inch above his ear and comb all that hair across the top, then part it again on his other side and comb all that hair across the other piece, then take some hair from the back and add that to it, and then spray it down heavily with a lacquer type hair spray! There is no way that we can cut the top even with the sides and leave it that long, therefore most barbers will simply not get involved in the top of this hairstyle. In my experience, customers who comb their hair like this in order to cover up a bald spot, do not want the barber to mess with it at all. We will usually just cut around the edges and leave the rest alone.

It's a good idea to let us know if you're *not* trying to cover the baldness and you don't mind it being short, because we will likely assume that you want to leave it long. Likewise, if you want it long, it's a good idea to let us know because some barbers might think it looks better short and take it upon themselves to alter it accordingly. It is my personal opinion that wearing it long does not make it look thicker. It only looks messier to me, but I would never cut the top short on a balding man without being sure that he wants it that way. Everyone has different tastes. We can't add hair to the bald spots. Like I said before, the barber's favorite style could very well be a mohawk, or a shaved head or something like that.

Most often, the men who are bald or in the process of going bald and only have a little hair in a ring above their ears just need their hair to be "trimmed up." That's really all they need to say for directions to most experienced barbers. It just means to clean it up nice around the ears and to taper the neckline and shave their neck.

Generally, barbers will cut the hair in the ears as part of the haircut without asking first. Some men don't like having their eyebrow hairs cut, so most barbers will ask first before trimming the eyebrows. I cannot understand why some men don't want them cut. There are some who hold the belief that if you cut them, they'll grow back longer or faster or thicker. This is a myth and is simply not possible. Cutting the end of the hair has no effect on the follicle, which is where it grows from beneath the skin. And they will never grow past a certain length anyway. I've never seen eyebrow hair growing down to a guy's shoulders.

Women And Girls

Most barber shops have at least one barber who will cut women's hair. Some barbers prefer not to. There are a lot of women who prefer to go to a barber for a short haircut, especially if they want no frills. If you are a woman and you want to get your hair cut in a barber shop, there are a few things you should be aware of. As I mentioned before, barbers typically don't fix the hair pretty after we cut it. We usually wet it with a spritz bottle or cut it dry. It's important that you come in with your hair clean, with no sticky styling products in it. Hair spray is the worst! When you add water to hair spray, it gets gummy and sticky. It's impossible to get a smooth pull with the comb, from the scalp to the point where we're going to cut it. It's impossible to do a perfect precision haircut with sticky stuff in the hair. If we absolutely have to, we will wash it, but we really don't want to spend the extra time to do that. Even though we charge extra for a shampoo, it's still not worth taking the extra time to do it. There are easier, faster haircuts waiting for us in the waiting room. The people waiting in the waiting room get impatient and sometimes leave if it looks as if it is going to be a long wait. It's not worth an extra $5.00 for the shampoo if a haircut walks out the door.

If you have long hair, you should brush all the tangles out before you get in the chair. When we do it, it takes more time and hurts more than when you do it yourself. Parents should brush young girls' hair to get the tangles out before they get in the chair too. It's really not fair to make the barber be the "bad guy." Most barbers don't mind doing a simple trim or basic medium length layer cut or short hair cuts on ladies. If you have a long layer cut or real thick hair, you really should go to a styling salon as it takes quite a bit more time to do.

If you do get your hair washed—whether you're in a barber shop or a salon—please don't lift your head up when we go to rinse the back. It's very common for people to do that. I guess they think it helps us to rinse the hair on the neckline. Your neck against the shampoo bowl is the only thing preventing the water from going down your back. If you lift your head, you will get a bath! It doesn't help us unless we're ready for it, in which case we will lift it or ask you to. You should keep your head all the way down on the shampoo bowl unless we lift it ourselves. Women are used to sitting in the chair facing the mirror. Barbers usually work with the customer facing away from the mirror. Once you have given the barber your instructions and you feel confident we've understood you correctly, you should trust that we're doing our best to do what you've asked us to do. If you keep asking, "You're not cutting it too short, are you?" or sticking your fingers in it while we're working, you're going to drive us nuts and we're not going to want to cut your hair again. Another reason we like to face the customer away from the mirror is because, if they are facing the mirror, they will turn their head to try to see what we're doing and it makes it uncomfortable for us to reach the hair. No matter how you turn your head or try to see it, there is no way you can see what we're doing in the back. If we finished one side and you did think it was too short, what would you do? Have us leave the other side longer and have a lop-sided haircut??? If you're having a complete panic attack, by all means, ask us to stop, say you've changed your mind and just want to leave. Otherwise, trust that we're doing what you told us to do and sit patiently. Please don't stick your fingers in your hair until we've gotten to the "rough draft" phase. We can always tweak things and make adjustments. It's not doing yourself any favors to be a pain in the butt.

Moms And Wives

Men frequently bring their wives with them to the barber shop. Maybe it makes him feel good to know she cares and he likes that. Perhaps he has no choice and she insists on it. He could be terribly embarrassed about it, but puts up with it anyway. Maybe he needs her to drive him there.

Often the wife will do all the talking, giving us the instructions as to how she wants it cut, and using terminology that's more applicable to women's haircuts. Men's haircuts are not "shingled" in the back. They are "tapered" in the back. It would seem to me to be quite humiliating to a man to just sit there while his wife tells the barber how to cut his hair. Unless he is really old, feeble, or blind, the rest of the shop is thinking how hen-pecked he is. As long as the man and his wife agree on the same haircut, it's not really a problem. Sometimes they are in disagreement which becomes a problem for us. We don't know who to listen to and we don't want to mediate. When we have a question, we don't know which one to ask. For example, "Do you want me to trim his eyebrows?" Should we ask her? Or him? Or what if we want to know if we should shorten his sideburns? Which one do we ask?

The other thing is that wives tend to want to stand over us and watch. I'm not sure if they're watching to make sure that we're doing it right or if they're watching to try to learn how to do it themselves, but it makes us nervous and aggravates us. Again … if it's more aggravating than it's worth to us, we will not want to do it every month.

If you are a wife who likes to go with your husband to the barber shop, or if you're a man who brings his wife with him to the barber shop, please make your instructions clear to the barber, and then the spectator should go sit down in the waiting area until we have a "rough draft" for them to come inspect. Please don't tell us it needs to be shorter on top if we haven't even gotten to the top yet. Just let us work until we get it to a certain point and then we can make adjustments.

Basically the same things apply to moms as to wives except that we assume the mom is in charge because she is the one paying for the haircut. Generally, we will listen to whoever is paying for the haircut. Mom's are notorious for asking the child if he wants more off the top before we've even touched the top in the first place. Wait until we get it to a certain point and then we'll ask if that's what you want.

When moms come in with several children, it's hard for them to keep their eye on all of them at the same time. The kids that are waiting always get bored. Kids usually won't read magazines or the newspaper. Some shops do have a TV though. The parent wants to relax and read a magazine and the kids are looking for trouble to get into.

There are two things that practically every child does in a barber shop, or will if their parents allow it. Every child wants to go over to an empty barber chair and pump it up and down and spin it around. They just can't resist it. I seriously doubt that most mothers would allow their child to pump and spin their eye-doctor's chair, or their dentist's chair, but for some reason, they usually just let their kids do it to our chairs and then *we* have to correct them. Even after we've corrected them, sometimes they'll keep doing it and the mom will say nothing. Our chairs are very expensive. We cannot allow children to play with them. Nor can we let them skate or dance around. It makes us nervous and is very distracting to the barbers. Often, kids will get right up under our counter behind the cords. We have sharp tools, mirrors and electric cords that are dangerous and could cause injury. The child could trip on the clipper cord while we're using it and cause us to make a mistake or cut someone. They could cause our tools or mirrors to fall on the floor and get broken. Children should never be allowed in our working area.

If there is a water cooler, every child wants to pour a cup of water. The usually pour it all over the floor and keep wasting it and creating a safety hazard. The parents should not allow their children to play like that. The barbers are trying to work. We are paying attention to the haircut we're working on. We don't have time to be watching your child and correcting them. That should be the parent's job. The person on whom we're working will become very nervous if they think we're not paying attention to what we're doing.

It's nice if a barber keeps something in the shop to entertain children. Toys or a television or children's books or something. Smart parents who bring more than one child should bring along something for their kids to play with. These days a cell phone or electronic games will do the trick. For older kids, a radio and earphones should work.

Confessions

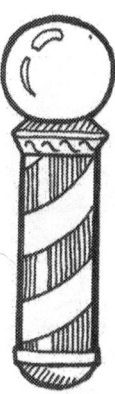

My Pet Peeves

I can only speak for myself, but I have sat around many barber shops discussing these situations with other barbers, and I feel that the majority would agree that the following situations all contribute to decreasing the odds of getting a good haircut and having an overall positive experience in the barber shop. These are things that might typically make a barber become surly.

—REPEATING INSTRUCTIONS: Once you give us the instructions, you should be able to trust that we didn't forget what you said. It's a bit annoying if you keep repeating yourself like we didn't hear you after we've already begun working on the haircut.

—CHANGING HORSES MIDSTREAM: Some people will give us instructions and then after we're halfway through they change their mind and tell us something different. Please stick to one haircut at a time.

—FINGERS IN HAIR: Please don't put your fingers in your hair until we are finished and have asked you to check it. If we're not finished yet, we cannot keep working with you wiggling around and flipping your hair with your fingers. This drives us nutty and increases the odds of injury.

—CHEWING GUM: Chewing gum while getting a haircut is not a good idea. When you chew with enthusiasm, your ears go up and down quite rapidly, making them a moving target, and increasing the chances of us cutting you. Chew with respect to the barber trying to work on you if you must chew gum while getting a haircut.

—ASKING US TO MAKE UP YOUR MIND: Sometimes people want to get their hair cut drastically shorter or drastically different than what they usually do, but they haven't made up their mind about it yet. So they will ask us what they should do. They want us to tell them what would look better. Our job is to do what you tell us to do and it's really not fair to push the responsibility off on us. What if we tell you to do something and then you hate it?

—FEET ON FLOOR: First of all, we're looking at the hair that we're cutting, not at our feet. I have tripped and almost fallen down many times, because someone's feet were on the floor in my way, and I trip over them. Secondly, people put their feet on the floor and then (whether they realize it or not) they move the chair around and back and forth, making themselves a moving target. Thirdly, we can't turn the chair the way we want it if a person's feet are on the floor. I've actually hurt my arm trying to turn a chair when someone's feet are on the floor.

—READING: It's ok to read, but you need to be aware of what you're doing. Flipping through the pages really fast makes your whole body move. Please turn the pages slowly and gently and be aware of your head moving. Watch that your newspaper or your elbow isn't in our way. Be careful that you don't tilt your head. If you need glasses to read, perhaps you should bring a magnifying glass. We're sorry if you can't read without them, but we have to have your glasses off to cut your hair. We can't work around them. Did you come to read or to get a haircut?

—MUMBLING/TALKING QUIETLY: If you want to have a conversation with us while we're cutting your hair, you need to speak loudly and clearly. We're in a shop full of other people talking, the radio or TV on, the clippers are noisy, blow-dryers are noisy, and most of the time we're standing behind you. Your voice projects straight ahead. If we're standing behind you and have the clippers on, we can barely hear you. We have to stop what we're doing to stand in front of you to hear what you're saying.

—SLOUCHING: If you're an especially tall person, or if the barber is a short person, it's very nice if you ask if they want you to slouch down in the chair to make it easier to reach. I'm quite short and often I have to ask guys to slouch down for me. *However*, the average sized person should sit straight in the chair. It's very important to sit with your rear end all the way back in the chair.

—ANIMATION: Some people talk with their hands. If you do that while getting a haircut, it will make your head a moving target. You really should keep hands, feet and objects under the cape and inside the chair at all times. When some people laugh real hard, they throw their head back. I cannot tell you how many times I've ruined a haircut because a guy threw his head into my clippers laughing. The clippers go right down to the skin halfway up the guy's head.

—SPECTATORS: If you bring a family member or friend along with you to get your haircut, please don't encourage them to stand right on top of us. Please ask them to wait in the waiting area. They are welcome to come inspect the haircut once we've gotten it to the rough draft phase. It makes most of us nervous to have someone watching us that closely, and often it causes the barber's hands to shake. It will increase the odds of getting a good haircut if the barber's hands are not shaking and they are not annoyed.

—EXPECTING US TO REMEMBER: It is entirely possible that your barber has cut somewhere around 700 haircuts since he saw you. If we've only cut your hair once or twice, it is unfair to assume that we will remember how we did it. We have people ask us if we were the one who cut their hair last. The customer only has to remember the barber's face in respect to a few other barbers in the shop. The barber has to try to remember the customer out of hundreds of other customers.

—THREATENING BODILY HARM: I have no idea what would make someone think that threatening their barber is a good idea. Maybe they are saying something in an attempt to be funny. Many times, a man will get in the chair and say something to the effect of: "If you cut my hair too short, my wife will come down here and break both of your legs." It does *not* increase the odds of getting a good haircut to threaten the person cutting your hair. It is a good way to make your barber surly and irritable.

—CONTROVERSIAL TOPICS: Please don't talk about controversial issues with us, such as politics, religion, wars, minorities etc. Even if you and the barber agree on the same things, there are other people in the shop who may or may not like what you're saying. We don't want people to be arguing nor do we wish to offend anyone. We also don't want our own personal views known to everyone in the shop. It's very hard for the barber to be agreeable if they feel strongly against what the customer is in favor of.

—SITTING CROOKED: When you are facing the mirror, look at yourself and the barber standing behind you. Look to see if your head is aligned with your body and in the middle of the chair. Don't cross your legs. Don't put your feet on the floor. Don't tilt your head to the left or the right. Don't look downward. It's very simple. Just sit straight and relax. We will adjust the angle of your head when we need to.

—LUNCHTIME: Barbers don't usually get a "lunchtime." We eat when we get a chance. We can't all eat at the same time unless we close the shop. We try to keep working as long as the shop is busy, but at some point we have to stop to get something to eat. Customers should patiently give the barber have at least ten minutes to gobble something down.

—WIGGLING: When you talk, don't nod or shake your head. Don't try to look at the barber's face. You can't have eye contact with us while we're working. Don't use your hands to talk. Try to keep the animation to a minimum. Don't fidget with the hair in your lap. Moving any part of your body, your hands, your feet or your legs makes your head move. Don't wiggle your knees back and forth. Try not to scratch your neck. Scratch if you absolutely can't stand it, but please warn us and don't do it repeatedly. Don't turn your head this way and that trying to watch what the barber is doing. If you have to sneeze, please try to warn us first.

—ANTICIPATION: There are people who are trying so hard to be helpful, that they will try to anticipate where we're going next, and move or angle their head in such a way as to give us what they must think is easy access to the area. If we're working in the middle of the back of their head, and they sense that we are moving to the right hand side of their head next, they will tilt their head to the left (head to shoulder tilt) before we get there. It's extremely annoying when people do this. I realize they are trying to be nice, but it does not help us in any way. It only causes us discomfort and aggravation. We would simply ask the customer or just push their head in that direction if we want it that way. It is best to sit with your head straight until otherwise directed.

—SLEEPING: It's very common for people to fall asleep while getting a haircut. It's relaxing and it feels good. We realize this. Most of us don't go out of our way to make it feel good, but it just does. It's flattering to us that you're so relaxed you can't stay awake, but please try not to go sound asleep. When people fall asleep sitting up in a chair, their head slowly goes down to their chest. Then they realize what they're doing and it startles them and they jerk their head up quickly. It's makes them move unexpectedly and causes the barber to jump, increasing the chances of cutting you or messing up the haircut. It's ok to relax and close your eyes. Just try to be careful of falling completely asleep.

—TELLING US WHAT TOOLS TO USE: It really is unfair to us for you to expect us to work the same way another barber or hairdresser does. We are all different. We all work in different ways and do things differently and with different tools. If you got a bad haircut form someone and they used the clippers on you, it doesn't mean the clippers are bad. The cutting tool doesn't make the haircut what it is. It's where we hold the hair with our comb or with our fingers that determines the length and the outcome of the haircut. Any sharp tool can cut the hair. It's not the tool's fault if it doesn't come out right.

—CLIPPER GUARDS: Most traditional barbers don't use the plastic guards and most cosmetologists don't use the Oster® clippers. The numbers of these two different tools do not correspond to the same length. A #2 plastic guard is not the same as a #2 metal "Oster" clipper blade. Be sure you know what you're talking about if you insist on a number, otherwise, it is best to describe your desired length by "short" "medium" "long" or by showing us with space between your fingers.

—DIRTY HAIR: Your hair doesn't need to be freshly washed, but it should be reasonably clean and free of sticky products. It's one thing if you didn't wash your hair for one day. That's no big deal to worry about. Three day old greasy hair is another thing. Some people wash their hair only once a week. No one wants to cut hair that is greasy or stinky. Barber shops don't usually wash the hair and only do so if we really need to or the customer really wants us to. It's also impossible to see if the haircut is blended properly on greasy hair.

—UNPLEASANT SMELLS: Some people think nothing of running to the barber shop for a haircut after they've been out fishing all day. Some come in after they've eaten a meal loaded with garlic and onions. Some people smoke and smell like cigars or cigarettes. Some bring babies in dirty diapers. We're working in close proximity to the customer. Bad smells are bad smells any way you look at it. Breath mints or cough drops work well for bad breath. I always use a breath mint after I smoke and before trimming a beard or mustache. Perfume or deodorants can help in a pinch. I always get a kick out of the guys who come in and say "I apologize, I'm all dirty and stinky." I always want to say back to them, "Oh, that's ok, I just ate some garlic and onion soup and I forgot to wear deodorant today." What do they expect us to say?

—PERSPIRATION: Many people come in sweaty and dirty, especially in the summer when it's hot outside. Parents pick their boys up at school where they've been playing on a playground and bring them straight to the barber shop. Some people have no air conditioning in their vehicle and come in all sweaty. Men come in after doing hard work in the heat. Sweat is not at all the same as water. A little damp is one thing, but wringing wet with perspiration is another thing entirely. It's impossible to do a good haircut on sweaty hair and it makes some of us nauseous and sick to our stomach to touch someone else's sweat. We have to see the hair dry in order to see the blend. Also, the clippers don't work well on wet hair. If you come in all sweaty, just go in the bathroom and rinse your face with water and use paper towels to soak up as much as possible. Sit in the air conditioning for a few minutes to cool down. Simply explain that you need a few minutes to cool down.

—HAIR PRODUCTS: It's impossible to do a precision, perfect haircut on sticky or slimy hair. Hair-spray turns into a yucky mess when you add water to it. At times, we want to wet it to cut it and it's so sticky, we can barely get the comb through it. Don't forget, we don't use a hairbrush to cut your hair. We use a fine-toothed comb. We insert the comb at the scalp and grab hold of the hair with our fingers, then follow through to the length where we want to cut it. We cannot get a nice smooth pull on the hair if it's sticky and it will take a lot more time to untangle. Not to mention, it's also very uncomfortable to the customer. And it's really gross to put our fingers into. Gel is just as bad, if not worse. Gel and hair-spray turn into a gross slimy "mush" when wet. It's difficult to see our guides, it feels gross in our fingers, it's slippery, it's uncomfortable for the customer and it costs us time. We have to take extra time to clean our tools thoroughly afterwards. Dunking a gel coated comb in the sanitizing solution doesn't work. We have to take the time to really clean it. It's like dropping a steak on the ground and then throwing it back on the grill, in that it still has dirt on it, but the dirt is sanitized. We understand that you have to use the product, but what's more important? You're going to wear this haircut for a month or so. Can you go one day without using your hair product so that you can get the best haircut possible?

—BED-HEAD AND HAT-HEAD: There are people who it seems roll right out of bed and go straight to the barber shop. You can see exactly in what position the guy slept with his head on his pillow. The hair is always smashed down in a swirl like a cowlick on whatever side he slept on. Sometimes even wetting it with water won't fix the problem. Some people don't like us to wet their hair. There's no way we can cut it perfectly if we can't get the hair to lie down to start with. If your hair is all smashed from the pillow and you're going to the barber shop, at least wet it and comb it. There are times when we just have to deal with it. But it's nice if you can make it a little easier on us. Sometimes guys come in after wearing a hat all day. We can cut it, but we tend to cut it until that ridge from the hat looks right and it might be shorter than you would normally wear it.

—CUTTING YOUR OWN HAIR: Everyone has a perfect right to right to cut their own hair and many people do. It looks so easy when they are watching us. Anything looks easy when someone is doing something they do every day of their life for many years. Skimming drywall looks simple when I watch my friend do it. He does it as a living every day. But I tried it once and it was very difficult to do. People attempt to cut their own hair and mess it up very badly sometimes. Then they come to us and expect us to fix it. The problem is that it is already too short in places. We cannot make it any longer. We can only make the long part shorter to make it even. We have to take it to the shortest point to make it even. We have to connect all the hair together. Otherwise there will be holes in the haircut and even an untrained eye can see an uneven haircut. Not to mention that the hair will not comb right or lay right if it is uneven. If you cut your own hair, and then come to us to fix it, expect it to be short and expect to live with it not looking right for a couple of months until the short parts grow out. And don't blame us for it.

—CLOSING TIME: If there are three barbers in a shop, and four customers walk in the door right before closing time, one of those barbers is going to be working a half hour or more past closing time. At some point, we have to just lock the door, and no amount of knocking on it or begging will get us to open it for you. If several customers come in at once, at the end of the day, we may lock up before the official closing time. Working men tend to come in right before closing time. We understand you have little choice, but please try (for your own sake as well as the barber's) to get there at least ten minutes before closing time. The barbers often have to pick up their own children from day care or after school care. We can't clean up the shop and close out the cash register until the last customer is finished. Often, all the barbers in a shop are stuck there until the last haircut is finished. As a single parent, I always had to pick my daughter up by 6:00 pm. Most day-care and after-school programs charge the parents $1.00 per minute they are late. Some parents have more than one child at two different schools to pick up. Most have families and like to be home for dinner. Some are moms and dads who have to be home to cook the dinner. If we have even one person waiting for a haircut at 4:45 (assuming 5:00 is closing time) we won't be leaving the shop until well after 5:30. It takes several minutes to do the haircut, several minutes to clean up our chair, several minutes to clean up the rest of the shop, and several minutes to take care of the money and get paid for the day.

—OPENING TIME: In every barber shop I've worked in, there are usually customers who come before the shop opens. They sit or stand outside waiting for the barbers to get there. The first barber to arrive at the shop has some things they need to do before they are ready to put a customer in the chair and start working. We have to turn on the lights and the air conditioner. We have to put the change money in the cash register and turn the sign on to "OPEN." We have to open the blinds, make a pot of coffee, etc. Each shop is different, but there are some things we have to do before we're ready to work. The customers should sit down in the waiting area until we call them to the chair. It seems bizarre to me, but most of the time, the first customer in line will go over to the barber's chair and stand there or help themselves and sit down in it. Some will even sit right on top of the cape, or grab it and hold it in their lap. Most of us are barely awake when we get to work. Some of us are parents who've been rushing to get their kids ready to go all morning. Some of us like to party at night and don't get enough sleep, then oversleep and rush to get to work on time. Sometimes traffic is bad getting to work during rush hour. Most of us don't arrive all happy and wide awake. Some folks can't function until they've had some coffee. Some barbers get to work early just so that they won't have to rush and they can get some coffee before the first customer arrives.

—CELL PHONES: It would really be nice if people would turn their cell phones off while getting their hair cut. We can't work around it unless you're on a walkie talkie and then the whole shop gets to hear your conversation. What do you do when you get your teeth cleaned? Or get an eye exam? We would appreciate the same courtesy you give to other service professionals. Most people should be able to let their calls go to their voice-mail for the time it takes to get a haircut. People seem to think nothing of answering their cell phone during their haircut. There is nothing we can do while you're on the phone. We have to just stand there doing nothing. We understand that it might be a very important call to you, but I don't think most people would answer their phones while in the doctor's chair, in the dentist's chair, eye doctor's chair, or lawyer's office! It's simply disrespectful to think the barber's time isn't as important. That's what voice mail is for. If you absolutely must answer your phone, at least try to make it quick. I've had people answer their phones and just start chatting away while I just stand there doing nothing. If there are other customers waiting, they get quite upset over the time being wasted, making them wait longer. One time, I had just opened up the shop and had four people waiting at the door. I was by myself as the other barbers had-n't gotten there yet. I was working on the first guy when he answered his phone and got quite involved in the conversation, leaving me standing there looking at the other customers, doing nothing. The other three customers were getting very agitated and shooting both he and I dirty looks. After about five minutes of just standing there, I took the next customer. put him in the other barber's chair, and started cutting his hair. I was halfway through when the first guy finally hung up his phone. I completed the second guy's haircut, and made the guy who was on the phone wait for me to finish him before I went back and finished his haircut.

Another time, I had a teenager to answer his phone during his haircut and start chatting with his buddy about what they were doing that night. I had been busy all day with no breaks and I was tired and I wanted a cigarette. There was no one else waiting in the waiting room. After about five minutes of him talking on the phone, I decided I might as well take advantage of the break and went outside and smoked a cigarette. I sat down and took my time.

—GETTING IN OUR CHAIR BEFORE WE CALL YOU: When we are finishing up with a customer, we're not ready to start the next one yet until the one we're working on has paid us and we've said "Thanks" and "Goodbye" to them. We need a minute to clean up our tools and our chair, and then we call the "next" customer. Often people will already be up and coming over to get into the chair when we're not finished with the one we're working on yet. We like to give each customer our full attention until we've said goodbye. Then we will give our next customer the same respect. Give us time to finish one before starting another. Think of it like a bank teller. You don't go up to the window until they call you. Some days are extremely busy and we don't get many, if any breaks between customers. The barbers try to sweep the floor between haircuts. If there are no breaks for any of the barbers, the hair clippings on the floor start getting pretty deep around the chairs. Not only does it look messy, but it is dangerous. The hair gets very slippery when you step on a thick patch and will make you go "skiing" across the floor. When it starts to get that heavy on the floor, one of the barbers should sweep the floor before calling a customer over.

Sometimes we need to use the restroom. If we've been working for several hours with no breaks between haircuts, we will just have to take a break and go.

Just like most other people, we like to eat lunch at a reasonable time. My hands shake when I'm extremely hungry and I get very grouchy and irritable. Often we may not get a lunch break till after 3:00. Sometimes we just can't wait that long and even if there are customers waiting, we have to just stop and take a quick break.

Some barbers smoke cigarettes. Anyone who has ever been addicted to nicotine knows what it feels like to have a nicotine fit. Some people's hands will even start shaking. A barber with shaking hands can potentially be dangerous, not to mention grouchy and irritable.

Many days we work for several hours before we finally get a little break. We have to make a choice between what's more urgent: sweeping the floor, smoking, going to the bathroom, eating or making an important phone call etc. We know that we might only get to do one of those things before another person comes in. We finally get to sit down for a second and a customer comes in and expects us to jump up and spring into action immediately. They have no idea it's the first time we've sat down all day and we're tired.

Physical health problems affect some barbers and there are some who are in pain after several hours of standing up working without any breaks. They may need a short break to take a pill or sit down for a few minutes.

On a busy day, we may run out of change in the cash register. One of the barbers has to drive to the nearest bank to get change.

There are times when one of the barbers may need to leave early or at a certain time for an appointment or something. It's best to just wait until the barber calls you to the chair.

—HEAD WOUNDS: There are people who will come in for a haircut the day after getting stitches in their head. People come in for a haircut the day after having skin cancers burnt off the heads, with the wounds still raw. I've had people come in with neck braces on and can't bend their neck. There are cuts and scrapes and bruises and all manner of wounds seen on men's heads in a barber shop. If it's a chronic or long term injury, then we just have to deal with it and do the best we can. Otherwise, it would be nice if people would wait a few days for the wound to heal a bit. First of all, sometimes it is really gross. I've seen wounds that have made me nauseous. Secondly, infections are often contagious.

The other thing is that people seem to expect it to be pain-free to get a haircut with a wound on their head! We have to lay the teeth of the comb firmly against a person's scalp in order to pick up the section of hair to be cut. There is absolutely no way around it. We also have to put a certain amount of tension on the hair. We pull it fairly taut from the scalp and if the scalp is sore, it's not going to feel good. The customer generally doesn't want us to skip that area of their head and leave that hair longer than the rest. But they will jump and act skittish and quite often will get an attitude with us like we're purposely hurting them! It's not our fault.

There is no way we can give you a perfect haircut if you have a wound on your head. The hair sticks to the moisture of the medicine, or the wound itself, and there is no way we can pull those hairs as tautly as the others.

Doctors are not known for the barbering skills. When a person gets stitches on their head the doctor will usually shave the area clean and then cut the surrounding hair real short. It's best to wait a couple of weeks or longer before expecting the barber to be able to fix it.

Sometimes customers want us to hide a scar on their head. There are two options. We can leave a large section of hair that doesn't connect evenly to the rest of the hair and is more noticeable than the scar itself, or we can leave all the hair long. It's like trying to hide a bald spot. In most cases, it brings more attention to the problem.

—ILLNESS: We find it annoying that people will come in for a haircut when they are obviously sick and contagious. We can't afford to be out of work and it leaves the shop short-handed if one of us gets sick. We don't get paid for sick days. We work in extremely close proximity to your face and we are touching you.

Some people will keep their child out of school because they are sick, and then bring them in for a haircut. Schools don't like it when children come to school sick, because colds and infections are contagious and it will spread all over the school. Sick children often cough right into the air while getting their hair cut, they wipe their nose with their hand and then touch the cape or something, and their germs are spread all over the place. Sometimes they even use the cape itself as a tissue to cough into or wipe their nose on. The barber can't stand far away and do a haircut on someone. We have to stand close to the customer. When we cut the bangs on a haircut, or do a mustache or beard trim, our face is right up close to the customer's face.

Because barbers don't get a retirement package, and typically get a small Social Security benefit, there are barbers in their 60's, 70's and even 80's still working. In general, elderly people don't fight illness as well as younger people do. I work with a barber right now who is diabetic and he has asthma. He has a lowered immune system because of all the medication he takes. He's 77 years old. If he knows someone is sick, he won't cut their hair. He will tell them to come back when they're well. He can't afford to get sick. If he could afford to stay home and not work, he would retire.

When one of us stays home sick with a cold or flu, it leaves the rest of the shop short-handed. It's very hard for the other barbers to work when we have to work short-handed. There is a lot of pressure on us to work as fast as we possibly can, because there are so many people waiting in the waiting room, and they will leave and go somewhere else if there is too long of a wait. We don't get time to go to the bathroom when we need to. We don't get time to eat lunch when we're hungry. We don't get time to smoke if we smoke. We don't get time to sweep the floor. We don't get time to go to the bank to get change. It's very stressful. We don't want to stay home and leave the shop short-handed because we care about the business and we know we will lose some customers if we do. We also care about our fellow barbers in the shop and we don't want for them to have to deal with the stress of working short-handed. We care about our job and don't want to disappoint the owner of the shop, and in some cases, risk being fired, by having to call in sick and making the boss have to scramble around trying to get whatever barber is off on that day to do us a favor and come in to work. No one wants to work on their day off. We all make plans for that time off that we need to run our lives. Sometimes the barber who is off on that day can't or won't come in. Sometimes they've made appointments that they can't re-schedule. We also have household duties and chores, grass to mow, laundry to do and all those things we have no time to do when we're working. There is not always the option of a replacement barber. It's a small business. We usually just have to deal with it and work short-handed. The sick barber knows it had better be serious before he stays home, because it will be hard on the barbers who are working on that day.

But the sick barber doesn't want to come to work being sick either, coughing and blowing our nose and talking in a hoarse voice. We don't want to get the other barbers sick and we don't to make our customers nervous of getting what we have. And we don't feel good and would rather stay home. It's very hard to work sick and we don't want to spread the illness around even more. We tilt our head downward all day long and it makes our nose runny. We have to quickly stop cutting the hair, put our tools down, rinse the hair clippings off our hands (or else we get a face-full of yucky hair clippings) and run to the bathroom quickly to blow our nose. We also have to use a tissue every time we cough. People would be grossed out if we cough into our hand and then put it back in their hair, or blow our nose and put our hands back in their hair, so we have to sanitize our hands in view of everyone before resuming what we were doing. This all takes time, is frustrating, and draws attention to the fact that we're sick, making everyone in the shop nervous that they're going to get it.

The barber that cuts the sick person's hair also takes the sick person's money which is germy and puts it in the register, then the other barbers and their customers touch the money.

Unless a person is getting married the next day or going to court or something of that nature, I cannot see where getting a haircut is something you have to do on any given day. It is not going to cause a person undue distress to wait three or four days for their cold to go away before getting a haircut and it would be much more considerate of other people.

About The Author

Mara's barbering career has spanned 25 years so far. She attended barber school away from home at the tender age of sixteen in 1980. She has worked her craft in many barber shops, both large and small, from Pompano Beach to Fort Pierce, Florida. She also lived and worked as a barber in Waldorf, Maryland. She was a barber school instructor at Roffler School Of Hair Design for several years. Because of her success, she has been instrumental in influencing many others including her husband and several friends and relatives, to learn the trade. Mara has owned and operated several barber shops in addition to managing several shops she's worked in.

About The Illustrator

Ellen Lyons Harris has been drawing since she could hold a pencil. After winning a number of awards in school, she answered her calling and chose to study at the prestigious Ringling School of Art and Design in Sarasota, Florida. She graduated Ringling with a B.F.A. and went on to study early childhood education and child psychology.

She has been a freelance artist for over twenty years and her work includes portraits, murals, logos and label design.

Ellen is an avid reader and writer and has written several childrens books. She also enjoys writing poetry, humorous prose and editorial essays.

When she is not piddling with pastels, paints or pushing a pencil, she enjoys wood working and furniture painting.

She lives in Florida with her husband, two children and two cats all of whom inspire her, none of whom are allowed in her studio when she is working.

If you would like to contact the artist for commission work you may do so at: ELyonsArt1@aol.com

978-0-595-42317-0
0-595-42317-5